The Architecture of the Superior Mind

How Genius, Talent, and Philistinism Shape Civilization, Power, and Human Progress

A Philosophical and Psychological Study of Genius, Talent, and Philistinism in their Relation to Human Society and its Struggle for a Better Social Order

The Architecture of the Superior Mind

How Genius, Talent, and Philistinism Shape Civilization, Power, and Human Progress

A Philosophical and Psychological Study of Genius, Talent, and Philistinism in their Relation to Human Society and its Struggle for a Better Social Order

(Illustrated, Refined & Edited)

By: Osias L. Schwarz and DD Editiorals

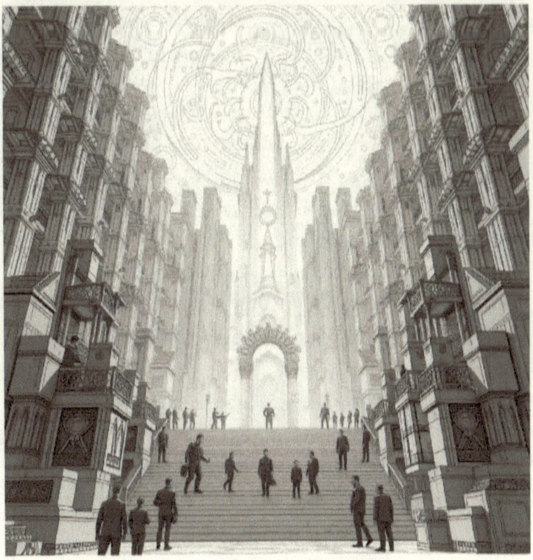

DD BOOKS
Publishers for New Generations

DD BOOKS
Publishers for New Generations

Publication Year: **2026** | Publisher: **DD Books**

ISBN: **9789372441741**

Edition: **First Edition, 2026** | Contact: ddsalesglobal@gmail.com

Book Name: **The Architecture of the Superior Mind: How Genius, Talent, and Philistinism Shape Civilization, Power, and Human Progress**

Author: **Osias L. Schwarz and DD Editiorals**

Price: **Rs 750/-**

Table of Content

Reader Note

This book is not a guide to success, nor a manual for ambition. It is something rarer and more demanding: a mirror held up to the human mind at its highest, lowest, and most conflicted states. The Architecture of the Superior Mind invites readers into a profound psychological and philosophical exploration of how people think, create, submit, rebel, and shape society—often without realizing the forces guiding them.

Across nine rigorously argued chapters, Osias L. Schwarz examines the differences between genius, talent, and philistinism—not as flattering labels, but as living mental structures that determine how individuals relate to truth, power, morality, creativity, and social order. This is a book about why some minds push civilization forward, why others resist change, and why most people remain trapped between fear and imitation. Readers will encounter ideas that are challenging, unsettling, and deeply illuminating. Schwarz dismantles comforting myths about intelligence, success, leadership, and adaptation. He shows that genius is not simply brilliance, but a costly form of inner freedom; that talent can flourish or stagnate depending on social conditions; and that philistinism is not stupidity, but a psychological defense against uncertainty, effort, and responsibility. The book reveals how societies reward conformity while punishing originality, how pseudo-superiority thrives in institutions, and why true creators are often misunderstood, exhausted, or crushed.

What makes this work especially compelling is its human honesty. Schwarz does not romanticize genius. He shows its fatigue, isolation, vulnerability to breakdown, and frequent conflict with social norms. At the same time, he exposes how mediocrity protects itself through custom, authority, and moral noise. Readers will recognize these dynamics everywhere—in politics, education, art, religion, workplaces, and even personal relationships.

Each chapter builds intellectual momentum while remaining rooted in lived experience: the struggle between instinct and idea, the tension between security and truth, the seductive danger of mysticism, the psychological cost of creativity, and the silent poisons that weaken collective thinking. This is not abstract philosophy removed from life; it is psychology that explains why societies stagnate, why revolutions fail, and why progress is always carried by a few at great personal cost.

For modern readers—especially those who think deeply, feel out of place, or question inherited beliefs—this book offers both recognition and challenge. It does not comfort; it clarifies. It does not flatter; it strengthens. It asks readers not merely to understand superior minds, but to examine their own habits of thought, fear, imitation, and courage. If you are drawn to psychology that explains power, creativity, conformity, and resistance with uncompromising clarity—this book will not merely interest you. It will stay with you.

Publisher's Note

In presenting The Architecture of the Superior Mind, the publisher recognizes both the intellectual weight of Osias L. Schwarz's work and the responsibility involved in bringing such a demanding text to contemporary readers. This edition is offered with deep respect for the author's original vision, argument, and critical spirit, while carefully shaping the presentation to ensure clarity, coherence, and accessibility for modern minds.

Schwarz wrote at a time when psychology, philosophy, and social criticism were inseparable disciplines. His work does not conform to today's simplified categories, nor does it soften its conclusions to suit prevailing comfort. Instead, it challenges readers to confront uncomfortable truths about intelligence, morality, creativity, and social organization. Our goal as publishers has been to preserve this intellectual integrity while making the text readable, navigable, and engaging for readers encountering it for the first time.

Language has been refined where necessary—not to alter meaning, but to restore flow and precision. Structural clarity has been enhanced to help readers follow complex arguments across chapters without losing the author's intensity or nuance. The result is an edition that remains uncompromising in content, yet far more approachable in form. This book matters today more than ever. In an age dominated by surface-level information, manufactured authority, and algorithmic conformity, Schwarz's analysis of genius, talent, and philistinism offers a powerful lens through which to understand contemporary crises of leadership, culture, education, and public thought. His critique of pseudo-superiority, institutional hypocrisy, and intellectual parasitism speaks directly to modern systems that reward visibility over substance and imitation over originality.

As publishers, we believe that classic psychological works must not be treated as museum artifacts. They must be reintroduced as living instruments of thought—tools that help readers understand themselves and the societies they inhabit. This edition aims to do precisely that: to invite reflection, provoke discussion, and restore depth to conversations about intelligence, creativity, and human progress.

We offer this work not as an easy read, but as an essential one. It is for readers willing to slow down, think carefully, and engage honestly. In preserving Schwarz's voice while easing entry into his ideas, we hope to make this book not only respected—but genuinely read, questioned, and lived with.

Introduction

Every civilization advances not because of its numbers, but because of a few minds that refuse to think as they are told. The Architecture of the Superior Mind is a journey into those minds—and into the psychological forces that oppose them.

This book explores one of the most enduring and dangerous questions in human history: why progress is rare, fragile, and resisted, even when its benefits are clear. Osias L. Schwarz approaches this question not through biography or ideology, but through psychology—examining how different types of minds relate to truth, power, fear, habit, and imagination.

At the heart of this work lies a stark distinction between three mental types: the genius, the talented individual, and the philistine. These are not social classes or moral labels, but psychological structures that shape perception, motivation, and action. Schwarz reveals how geniuses create new paths of thought at immense personal cost, how talent often adapts to existing systems, and how philistinism preserves itself through imitation, authority, and resistance to effort. Readers are led through an intellectual landscape that includes creativity and exhaustion, originality and misunderstanding, clarity and mysticism, courage and conformity. The book examines how societies treat their most original thinkers, why institutions favor pseudo-superiority over real insight, and how fear disguises itself as tradition, morality, or common sense. One of the book's most powerful contributions is its analysis of mental health and creativity. Schwarz challenges the notion that genius is inherently pathological, showing instead that breakdown often results from overexertion, social hostility, and the burden of pioneering thought. He distinguishes between productive originality and regressive mysticism, between deep speculation and intellectual decay, offering readers tools to recognize clarity amid confusion.

Throughout, the tone remains unsentimental and precise. This is not a celebration of genius for its own sake, nor a condemnation of the average person. It is a serious inquiry into how human potential develops—or fails—under specific psychological and social conditions.

For modern readers navigating a world saturated with noise, performative intelligence, and manufactured authority, this book offers something rare: intellectual grounding. It teaches how to recognize substance beneath appearance, how to resist mental passivity, and how to understand the true cost of thinking independently.

This is not a book to skim. It is a book to engage with slowly, argue with, return to, and reflect upon. Those who do will find themselves better equipped—not merely to understand superior minds—but to question the structures that shape their own thinking and their society's future.

Chapter-1.
Genius and Talent: How Great Minds Think, Create, and Transform

This chapter explores the hidden architecture of exceptional minds—how genius differs from talent, and why certain individuals reshape knowledge, culture, and moral horizons. By examining patterns of perception, creativity, memory, and motivation, it reveals not merely how great minds think, but how their inner lives become engines of transformation for humanity itself.

General Characteristics of their Fields of Activity

A person of talent brings individual cases and isolated phenomena under an already known rule or law. A person of genius, by contrast, moves in the opposite direction: from a small number of special cases or isolated facts, he rises toward a new general rule, a new law.

Yet the creation of new generalizations is not the sole domain of genius. Sagacity does not show itself only in discovering something entirely new. It is equally required in reducing the unknown to the known, the apparently known to what is truly unknown; in identifying connections between things commonly regarded as unlike, as well as in separating and discriminating things that are vulgarly assumed to be identical. Genius lies in discovering relationships between events and ideas that seem wholly unrelated to the talented person, and in giving clear expression or concrete realization to what, in others, exists only as vague, hesitant, and groping feelings or wishes.

From a maximum of observations, the person of talent draws a minimum of conclusions; the genius, on the other hand, draws a maximum of conclusions from a minimum of observations. Talent is chiefly concerned with applying, interpreting, modifying, and verifying the creations of genius.

The striking novelty of the genius's creations is largely due to the fact that he draws material for his reasoning and for his mental life as a whole from every available source. He is unhampered by prejudice or by fear of consequences. Unlike the merely talented person, he does not rely solely on the limited stock of accepted scientific knowledge or on those conscious personal experiences that enjoy social approval. He also draws upon facts and claims that are tabooed, unpopular, or obscure, as well as upon the vast store of subconscious perceptions and long-forgotten memories.

Here the genius must be clearly distinguished both from the philistine and from the so-called psychic medium. The philistine, dulled by routine and mental inertia, occasionally resorts to stimulants, intoxicants, or excitements in order to break, for a brief moment, the barriers between the subconscious reservoir and the dried-up streams of conscious thought. Psychic mediums—hypnotic subjects, crystal-gazers, clairvoyants, mind-readers, and the like—when not relying on fraud, seek artificially induced states of mental dissociation, inner absorption, or hypersensitivity, in order to extract from the subconscious forgotten trivial memories or perceptions obtained directly or by suggestion.

The genius, by contrast, draws naturally, steadily, slowly, and effortlessly, and always in his normal state, upon the valuable contents of his subconscious mind. He does so by keeping the gates of consciousness permanently open and by holding his attention firmly upon some vital question or problem. Just as he draws fearlessly, patiently, and impartially upon this vast but chaotic inner store, so he refuses to dismiss from consciousness any thought, feeling, or impulse that claims his attention before it has found its proper place or function in his mental economy. No matter how distasteful, unflattering, tabooed, or socially unacceptable such inner material may appear, he subjects it to honest scrutiny.

If, for any reason, he is compelled to relegate certain thoughts to the subconscious, he never allows them to remain there long in an isolated, erratic, or dissociated state. Left unattended, such fragments may develop into mental weeds—fixed ideas, phobias, obsessions, delusions—which tend to overrun, distort, or even break up the normal personality.

The phenomenon of heightened memory in fever, dreams, or trance states shows that subconscious or automatic mental activity—subconscious perception and memory—is richer in content, receptivity, and inventive power, but poorer in order, harmony, organization, selection, adaptation, and purposeful use than conscious mental activity. Conscious perception, memory, and judgment are more truly our own.

Conscious mental activity consists in selecting, from among our countless present, past, and possible impressions, those that can be organized into a working system in accordance with our dominant guiding ideas and ideals. In an average, healthy consciousness there is little room for ideas that do not fit into such a purposeful scheme. These ideas are soon forgotten at the conscious level, even though verbal or nominal traces may linger for a time.

Conscious activity is never a mere repetition of past activity; it is always selective, critical, and goal-directed. It tends toward harmony and purpose. Semi-conscious, inspirational, or spontaneous activity departs even further from the usual patterns, yet it is not consciously goal-directed for the actor himself. Automatic behavior, on the other hand, is an almost exact repetition of earlier actions; it may aim at a goal, but one that is unknown in advance to the person performing it.

The fact that careful observation can always distinguish between truly conscious and merely seeming conscious activity proves that consciousness is not a passive by-product or a simple mental image. It is a regulating force: helpful in new situations, though often disturbing in familiar ones. To be conscious means to be influenced by, to influence, and to harmonize with the total life of the mind.

The achievements of talented individuals are conscious, anticipated, mildly original, and voluntary. The creations of genius are semi-conscious, inspirational, spontaneous, and profoundly original. The average person is best suited for muscular or automatic activities.

The convictions of the genius are chiefly first-hand. They are drawn directly from the hard discipline of personal experience, from the social and cosmic environment, and they are deeply rooted in the innermost core of his being. Talented people, and especially average individuals, tend to adopt the opinions of others wholesale. They do not clearly separate fact from interpretation or emotional valuation, whereas the genius extracts the objective elements of facts and adds his own interpretation and evaluation only where necessary.

The intellectual seeds planted in the average or talented mind either perish or develop into thoughts closely resembling their original form.

The genius, however, grafts his own thoughts and feelings onto what he receives, thereby producing new and improved intellectual growth. Through this process, he invents means of increasing truth, beauty, love, and social happiness, and of enriching and ennobling human life.

Difference of Degree

Does the person of genius differ from the average person merely in degree, or in kind—in quantity or in quality? And how does he differ from the person of talent?

The answer depends on the standpoint from which we observe them. What appears as a quantitative difference from the objective point of view appears as a qualitative difference from the subjective point of view.

The abilities of the original person do not differ in kind from those of the routine individual; they differ only in degree. They are more fully developed and yield richer results. Viewed from above, from a strictly philosophical standpoint, the genius may appear little more than an average person. Yet from the social and human perspective, the quantitative difference is so great that it may rightly be taken as a difference in quality. If we examine abilities alone, geniuses differ from others only in degree; but if we consider their achievements and their fields of activity, the difference becomes one of kind.

All mental processes—perception, memory, imagination, judgment, reflection, and their various combinations—presuppose and arise from a fundamental dualism: between the self and the not-self, the present and the past, the present and the future, the actual and the possible, the known and the unknown. These processes share this basic structure and rely on the same elementary operations of discrimination, identification, and connection. They differ only in the degree of complexity involved and in the distance between the related facts.

What holds true for the various mental processes within a single individual also applies when comparing the genius with the average person. The genius possesses no mental abilities that are absent in the average individual; he merely possesses them in greater abundance. Where the mental energy of the ordinary person is quickly exhausted when dealing with simple, concrete facts related to everyday needs, the genius can apply his mental energy with equal ease to abstract ideas and to vast complexes of facts that have no immediate relevance to narrow practical interests.

Aim and Ability

Ability and aim, force and direction, are inseparable. This does not mean that the same ability must always move in the same direction, or that it cannot be redirected toward a different aim. Nor does it mean that the same aim cannot be pursued by different abilities. The number of possible aims and directions of activity is unlimited, but the number and magnitude of our abilities, energies, and impulses are limited. From this arises the necessity of neglecting, reducing, or subordinating certain aims in favor of others.

The very act of becoming interested in a particular line of activity and beginning to pursue a specific aim often reduces—frequently without our awareness—our ability to pursue other aims. Aims and means lie along the same line; only the means must be traversed before the aim can be reached. Because this is often the only distinction between them, a means may become an aim, and an aim may in turn serve as a means toward a further end.

Some geniuses differ from one another more in their aims than in their abilities, as seen among various classes of scientists—physicists, chemists, geologists—or among artists—poets, novelists, dramatists, painters, sculptors, musicians, and actors. Others differ more in ability than in aim. Observers, scientists, and philosophers alike seek truth; yet the first remain with facts and simple relations, the second rise to more complex relations and concrete concepts, and the third ascend to the most general concepts, to comprehensive worldviews and first principles.

Philistines differ from geniuses in both aims and abilities. The talented individual differs from the genius within the same field more in ability than in aim. What is for the genius a mere means or secondary aim becomes, for the less able person working in the same direction, a primary aim. Conversely, what serves as a primary aim in one field or for one class of genius or talent may be only a secondary aim or a means for another.

Natural Interests

Beyond differences in ability, further fundamental distinctions between genius, talent, and the average mind must be sought in the quality and quantity of their innate, natural interests. These interests determine the content and direction of consciousness, perception, memory, imagination, reverie, and thought; they activate and stimulate mental abilities.

We notice and remember spontaneously, involuntarily, and easily what directly interests us. We attend to and remember deliberately, intentionally, and slowly what interests us only indirectly. Whatever runs counter to our natural interests and inclinations is disregarded or pushed out of consciousness.

To the philistine, matters such as food, shelter, clothing, romantic affairs, bodily appearance, gossip, external approval, material possessions, and superficial intellectual pleasures are just as serious and central to life as the pursuit of abstract and impersonal knowledge, beauty, social reform, social happiness, self-perfection, self-approval, spiritual wealth, and refined intellectual joy are to the genius. The philistine is no less insatiable, persistent, or even inventive in trivial pursuits than the genius is in lofty aspirations. The difference lies in the outcome: the philistine's insatiability harms society as a whole, and his craving for novelty consists merely in a love of sensations, fashions, appearances, and distinctions.

A philistine would feel just as unhappy if forced to eat the same food every day and wear the same clothes for a year as a philosopher would feel if compelled to think the same few thoughts repeatedly or to read only one book throughout life. The person of talent stands midway between the genius and the average individual. The pseudo-superior person, or the ordinary person of action, adds to philistine and sham intellectual pursuits a striving for power, influence, popularity, and political or economic leadership. The semi-superior person combines some genuine intellectual pursuits with these ambitions.

Once an individual's natural interests are given, the characteristic objects of his thought, the enduring content of his consciousness, and his typical modes of action follow as necessary consequences, for whoever wills the end also wills the means.

An intense and exclusive interest in a particular object, combined with limited ability, can accomplish more in that direction than great ability guided by weak interest. Judged solely by results, such a person—driven by one-sided desire and perseverance—may be mistaken for a genius. This is especially true of financial magnates, political or military heroes, and explorers. True genius, however, is more or less universal. It produces many-sided results in a relatively short time, with comparatively little labor, simple tools, little premeditation, and without a perseverance that is consciously fixed on a narrow aim.

Self-Instruction

In study and self-education, the genius seeks confirmation rather than stimulus for his creations, whereas the talented individual seeks impulse and stimulation for mental activity.

Some people learn in order to know; others read merely to have something to talk about. A third group uses learning for theoretical or practical ends, including intellectual or financial speculation. Both extremes—the disinterested genius and the selfish materialist—belong to this third group. Dilettantes, casual readers, and many professors belong to the second, while scholars and serious readers belong to the first.

For the truly superior person, one who possesses a genuine hunger for knowledge, books serve to supplement, complete, broaden, and unify knowledge gained through personal experience. From books he seeks stimulation for further thought and observation; they widen his intellectual horizon and make his mind more receptive to an ever-expanding range of impressions. They help him overcome, at least in imagination, the limitations imposed by daily routine, the struggle for livelihood, and the brevity of human life. Through books he becomes acquainted with people, events, and eras inaccessible to direct observation.

To him, book knowledge is not—as it is for the pseudo-superior person—a substitute for communion with people and nature, an excuse for laziness, or a burden to be stored and displayed. It is indispensable nourishment for the mind, to be digested, assimilated, and transformed into living energy—into dynamic, guiding ideas. Unlike the rigid scholar who is absorbed solely in the opinions of others, the genuinely superior mind prefers to consult life directly and to remain in living contact with it.

Genius and Erudition

In science, the conservative element is represented by scholars and savants; in practical life, it is often represented by women. The more we know the opinions of others, the fewer opinions of our own we are able to form. Vast erudition is frequently accompanied by narrowness of outlook. The memory of the purely scholarly mind becomes swollen with verbal knowledge and with carefully learned expressions of praise or admiration for achievements of the past, while its mental vision remains blind to the living movements of progress and to the intellectual ferment taking place all around it.

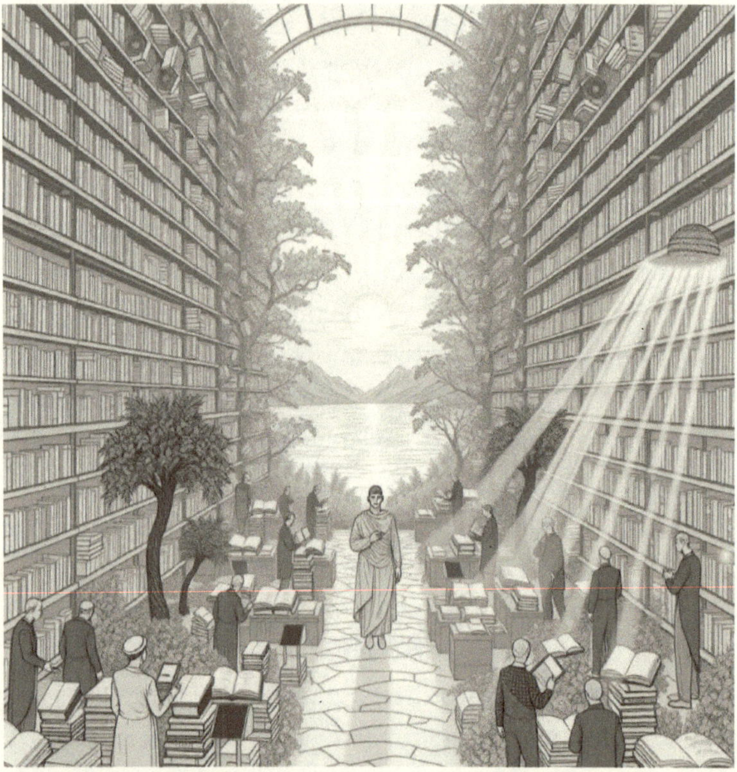

Erudition, beyond a certain limit, becomes an obstacle to originality. For the original mind, learning is only a means, never an end in itself. In the works of others, the genius seeks not so much information as stimulation for his own creative activity.

Memory

The memory of the genius is assimilative; that of the savant is chiefly reproductive. The genius retains experiences that can be integrated into his own original inner content, creating harmony and meaningful connections.

The memory of the scholar and of the average individual, by contrast, is largely chronological and accumulative, except in the narrow sphere of personal interests or professional specialization.

The genius remembers what he understands; others may, in time, come to understand what they have memorized. Excessive memorization—the absorption of intellectual material not demanded by an organic inner need—usually obstructs true digestion, assimilation, and understanding.

Imitation and Teachableness

Just as the human infant appears disadvantaged by helplessness and clumsiness when compared with animals born equipped with instincts for self-preservation, so the genius often appears awkward, backward, unteachable, unsociable, or poorly adapted when compared with the philistine or the pseudo-superior person, who quickly learns to imitate the language, manners, and outward forms of others.

Yet the initial advantage of animals—their fixed inherited instincts—later becomes an obstacle to learning from experience and to further development. In the same way, the apparent teachableness of the philistine, his passive adaptability and inborn imitativeness, becomes a barrier to genuine self-education, creative adaptability, and inner growth.

The genius may lack skill in the worship of tradition, routine, and convention; but the philistine is helpless when confronted with innovation, self-directed learning, or broad and unfamiliar problems.

Imitation is the most natural and easiest method of mental growth for the philistine and for one-sided or semi-superior individuals. Learning begins with the imitation of outer form—

words, appearances, conventions—and only gradually, if at all, proceeds toward assimilation of the hidden inner meaning.

The development of the genius moves from within outward—from thought and feeling toward expression. This explains his difficulty in imitation and his awkwardness when he attempts to speak or act without genuine conviction. It explains why actors are rarely great playwrights, and why playwrights seldom excel as actors. Even a many-sided genius may seem less adaptable and less teachable than semi- or pseudo-superior individuals.

In the philistine and the pseudo-superior person, form and content are often dissociated; form becomes an end in itself. In the genuinely superior mind, form and content are inseparable. He cannot accept one without the other. He cannot speak merely for the beauty of sound, nor act simply to please or to imitate. He cannot publicly adopt noble forms while secretly pursuing ignoble ends, as the pseudo-superior person often does. Where the philistine needs only to adopt a form, the genius must also assimilate the content concealed within it—and this inevitably slows his learning from others.

While the philistine and the pseudo-superior person are satisfied with superficial assimilation, the genius is compelled to penetrate to the origin and ultimate consequences of ideas. He follows thoughts back to their remotest causes and forward to their furthest implications. This depth of inquiry explains his apparent slowness. The seeming quickness and adaptability of pseudo-superior individuals rests on superficiality, lack of intellectual conscience, and purely verbal learning. They are richer in words than in ideas, richer in appearance than in reality. The reverse is true of the genius. Like an infant, he possesses more states of consciousness than words with which to express them. The philistine, by contrast, is poor in both ideas and expression.

Thought-Pride, Verbosity, and Grandiloquence

Just as great wealth diminishes the subjective value of money for the millionaire, so the abundance of ideas diminishes the subjective importance of any single thought for the genius. There is pride of thought as there is pride of wealth. Verbosity and grandiloquence betray intellectual pride and often conceal inner barrenness. They substitute inflated language for genuine thought. Verbosity also signals confusion of ideas and an inability to separate what is clear and valuable from what is vague and useless. Genuine genius and verbosity never coexist. The truly original mind becomes almost indifferent to intellectual pleasure; ideas arise naturally and effortlessly, without conscious struggle. Lacking the experience of painful intellectual labor, such a mind cannot savor the dramatic joy of conquest that delights the intellectually poor.

Superior and Average Mind: Social Significance

Action precedes reaction; spontaneous activity precedes voluntary action; play precedes serious work. Reverie, imagination, and hypothesis come before the discovery of new facts and realities. Serious activity is merely play transformed and directed by unsatisfied needs. Facts are often nothing more than verified and modified hypotheses, just as reaction is action reshaped by external influence.

Reaction is never equal to external action; it is only proportional to it. No external stimulus could provoke a response if the individual were not already active from within. Facts do not force themselves upon the mentally inert; education, reasoning, and argument do not move the philistine masses. Insults do not readily provoke those free from vanity, unless they strike directly at the instinct of self-preservation.

Children, women, and the wealthy—whose needs are largely met by others and who are kept at a distance from the harsher struggles of reality—can afford to indulge in play, reverie, illusion, incomplete perceptions, and unverified hypotheses. Adults, men, and the poor, by contrast, are compelled to rely on their own resources. They must therefore control and direct their activity, test their assumptions, and bring them into conformity with reality. The philistine masses, though prone to superstitions, mystical beliefs, illusions, and prejudices concerning distant people and matters that do not directly or immediately affect them, would be crushed by reality if they failed to form reasonably accurate judgments about the people and things that constitute their immediate environment.

The philistine sees in people and objects little more than what he already anticipates—and he anticipates very little. He does not perceive new facts unless they are simultaneously forced upon him by the pressure of immediate circumstances and by the initiative of geniuses.

If the genius appears more deeply impressed by the same influences that act upon everyone, it is because he is more disinterestedly active, because he anticipates more, and because he is always ready to meet people and events halfway. Unlike the philistine, he does not squander his energy on petty, trivial, or selfish concerns.

Human beings are far more capable of sustained, serious activity than animals precisely because, owing to prolonged infancy, they possess a richer store of play activities to draw upon in moments of crisis. Human intelligence confronts needs and obstacles more effectively because it remains active even in their absence—before they arise and after they have passed.

The genius solves the broader, future-oriented problems of life more successfully than the philistine because his momentary, personal, selfish, and bodily interests are reduced to a reasonable minimum and therefore do not absorb his entire attention and energy.

Just as it is not the total relative weight of the brain, but rather the greater development and complexity of the frontal and parietal lobes, that distinguish the genius from the philistine, so—in terms of energy—it is not greater total vitality or even greater mental force that characterizes the genius. What distinguishes him is the surplus of mental energy available for higher, synthetic, conceptual, general, disinterested, and prospective thinking. This surplus arises because the genius expends only a minimal amount of energy on lower, particular, personal, and immediate interests.

It is easier to impart motion to a body already in motion than to one apparently at rest, for in reality there is no true state of zero velocity. A body at rest adheres ever more closely to its surroundings, acquiring a kind of negative inertia that must be overcome before movement can begin. In the same way, intellectual movement is easily imparted to a thinking individual, but not to the adult philistine who has not progressed beyond childhood inertia and who clings ever more firmly to fixed dogmas, superstitions, and customs of his immediate social environment, developing an increasing aversion to free and independent thought.

The genius represents the dynamic, progressive element of the animate world. He cannot take root permanently anywhere. He moves freely—at least mentally—from one social class, nation, or race to another; from present to past and future; from one object of thought to another. For this reason he is disliked by the philistines, who form the static, conservative, and often regressive element of society. The genius recalls them from the easy downward path and urges them along the difficult upward course of human development.

A genius functions as a social organ whose task is to elaborate a new ideal or aspiration, to be balanced and completed by the ideals created by other geniuses. Despite the many-sided symmetry of the social organism, geniuses of the same class cannot readily replace one another, for each possesses something uniquely his own, even in relation to others of the same type. The average person, by contrast, represents a mere social unit or cell—easily replaceable and frequently misplaced owing to social imperfections—thereby hindering the proper functioning of the social organism and of its creative organs.

Moral geniuses form the brain, the cerebral center, of society. Agitators, organizers, and leaders constitute its nervous system: they transmit to the moral geniuses detailed information about social disorders, give the alarm when institutions malfunction, and convey to the philistine masses—who represent the muscular system—the general remedial measures devised by the moral geniuses. Other geniuses—technical, artistic, scientific, or philosophical—perform particular functions but are not primarily concerned with the welfare of the whole organism. Moral geniuses alone ensure that these specialized functions proceed normally and are not diverted into parasitic channels, whether within or outside society.

Just as in the individual organism it is not the nerves that feel pain or determine its causes and remedies, but the brain, working silently and unseen, so in society it is not the pure agitators or mere truth-tellers who fully grasp the suffering of humanity or elaborate adequate remedies. This work is done by the obscure, solitary, and often unnoticed moral geniuses. The pure truth-teller reports injustices, oppression, and intolerance without fully comprehending their depth, causes, or consequences. The pure agitator arouses the masses to action without fully understanding the urgency, scope, or authorship of the message he delivers.

As social evolution shows signs of moving away from extreme specialization toward a more democratic order—in which differentiation is transferred to tools, institutions, and machinery rather than to human beings—it is natural to encounter individuals who combine intellectual or artistic genius with moral insight, producers who are also distributors of ideas, and moral geniuses capable of carrying their own messages to the people. We may even find agitators who genuinely feel and partly formulate the truths they proclaim, and dramatists who can enact their own creations.

What should surprise and trouble us is the opposite: actors who distort an author's meaning because they cannot feel as he does; agitators who make a profession of transmitting messages of hope while remaining vain, selfish, and incapable of self-sacrifice; interpreters who misrepresent the teachings of geniuses. It should pain us that the masses have been so degraded by systems of exploitation as to lose the capacity to understand the calm expression and inner logic of the moral genius, and therefore require the noise, declamation, and gesticulation of the mere agitator to be shaken from their mental torpor. The superior individual—that is, the person of great talent—possesses not only a more varied and heterogeneous impressibility but also a more highly developed consciousness than the average person. His consciousness is more selective and purposeful, more differentiated and discriminating, more orderly, harmonious, economical, and adaptive. It is more spontaneous, more self-active, and qualitatively richer—richer, above all, in aims and interests.

The average person lives largely a subconscious, suggestible, and imitative life. Only when confronted with unfamiliar or unexpected circumstances does he become self-conscious. Once the storm of novelty has passed, his mind sinks back into the comfortable habitual slumber of a semi-conscious, almost hypnotic existence. In the normal superior individual, the opposite is true: his self-conscious personality is steadier, more persistent, and more continuously awake.

The average individual is both hetero-suggestible and auto-suggestible. His ideas can be brought into harmony only under the influence of some external authority. Left to himself, his mind falls into disorder, disharmony, and submission to fixed ideas and false beliefs. The superior person, by contrast, is cosmically and socially suggestible: his ideas harmonize with one another under the guidance of real, objective relations. Blind imitation of local, self-appointed authorities accounts for the overwhelming majority of ordinary people's thinking, feeling, and acting. This fact explains why statistical methods are of such limited value in psychology and the social sciences.

The personality of the original individual is concentrated and shaped primarily by inner forces rather than by external circumstances. Changes in material conditions, domestic life, nationality, race, or profession do not deeply affect his inner core. The personality of the inferior individual, on the other hand, is diffuse and scattered, held together largely by external pressures. Once these pressures are removed, the inner core quickly dissolves.

When educated philistines—and especially pseudo-superior individuals—seek eagerly to live among, or be associated with, a so-called higher social class, they do so not merely to deceive others about their worth. They are also driven by their own suggestibility and imitative tendencies, which make them feel and become different in different environments. Only the genuinely superior individual, endowed with a strong and original personality, can mix freely with all social groups without losing anything of his inner value. On the contrary, he gains in breadth and consistency. By defending his convictions—openly or within his own inner forum—against those of others, he learns which elements of his character possess lasting social value and which are not worth preserving or transmitting to the future. In general, the average person possesses less discriminative power, less spontaneity, and less inner mobility than the genius; laypersons less than specialists; women less than men; animals less than humans; plants less than animals; and inanimate matter less than living substance. The philistine accepts almost without selection the opinions and sentiments imposed by authority. He scarcely chooses his spouse, friends, vocation, or sources of pleasure and information; he associates with those whom chance places around him; his horizon rarely extends beyond the narrow circle into which circumstances have thrown him. He submits passively to the existing order, incapable of imagining a better one.

His personality is so little his own—so weakly rooted in inner spontaneity and so dependent on immediate social pressures—that it disintegrates under one or two years of solitary confinement, yet remains intact under a lifetime of monotonous labor. The degree of solitude a person can endure, and the inverse degree of monotony, blind obedience, and enforced sociability he can tolerate before becoming distressed, may therefore serve as a measure of his individuality, originality, and inner independence.

The average civilized individual fears nothing more than solitude, exclusion, or the relaxation of external pressures. Deprived of these supports, his unstable and hysterically predisposed mind threatens to fragment, to run wild, or to collapse into incurable mental disorder. His apparent willingness to obey masters, to serve as a tool, his unthinking opposition to movements aimed at his emancipation, and his tendency toward hero-worship all arise from this fear of inner disintegration.

External pressures, imposed by exploitative systems, prevent the average person's mind from developing and instead fragment it into incoherent impulses. Ironically, the same pressures that destroy his inner unity become necessary to maintain his outer, artificial stability.

The less one possesses inwardly, the more one seeks to possess outwardly. The less ability one has, the more noise one makes about one's supposed merits. The less reason one has for genuine pride, the more one boasts of ancestry, family, friends, institutions, professions, parties, possessions, or social rank. Those who have profited least from education are often the proudest of their schools and titles.

In the social realm, the philistine resembles an inert body in the physical world. Like such a body, he does not enter intellectual or moral activity spontaneously; he requires an external impulse. Nor does he abandon beliefs, customs, or moral practices imposed by past authorities—even when they have become harmful—until driven in another direction by a new external force.

The spontaneity of the genius resembles that of an explosive substance: it does not require an external cause proportional to its effects. What appears as sudden spontaneity is in fact the culmination of countless small, accumulated influences that become visible only with the addition of one final, seemingly decisive stimulus.

The essential difference between the philistine and the genius lies in this: in the former, external influences remain isolated, unconscious, and ineffective; in the latter, these same small, impersonal social and cosmic influences are gathered, integrated, and transformed into new thoughts, feelings, and acts of will—personal, powerful, and capable of influencing others.

Difference in Thinking

The thinking of a superior individual differs from that of the average person in one fundamental respect. Once a train of thought has begun in the superior mind, it tends to persist even after the original stimulus has ceased. It spreads beyond immediate experience to include past and possible experiences. In the average mind, by contrast, thought is brief, limited in scope, and evoked only by immediate external stimuli.

For the genius, thinking is an organic and enduring necessity—an end in itself. For the philistine, thinking is either a casual and aimless play activity or a mere instrument used only under pressure to satisfy urgent bodily needs.

Under normal conditions, the philistine neither cares for nor is capable of sustained reflection on general problems—such as the origin, meaning, and aim of life or the universe—unless driven by intense psychological pain or deep dissatisfaction. Even then, his thinking rarely progresses far beyond the mere formulation of questions. In the genius, however, the organ of thought—shaped by hereditary tendencies and spontaneous variation—has become permanent and self-sustaining. It functions under the slightest inner stimulus, and even in the absence of pain or surplus energy, transforming thought into a continuous and vital activity of the mind.

The genius is able to distinguish, within any object or phenomenon, what is typical, general, essential, and enduring from what is individual, particular, accessory, and changeable. The philistine, by contrast, tends toward one of two extremes: he either treats every object and event as wholly unique and incomparable, or else he regards everything as uniformly typical. The person of talent and the scientist are less penetrating and therefore more cautious than the genius. They require the observation of many similar instances before daring to separate the essential from the accidental.

The philistine, like the child and the primitive human being, confuses fable with fact, second-hand knowledge with first-hand experience, accident with essence, form with spirit, the fleeting with the eternal, means with ends, copies with originals, tautologies with explanations, particulars with generals, the artificial and conventional with the natural, the changeable with the permanent, the trivial with the important, the local with the universal, appearances with reality, and words with things, thoughts, feelings, or acts of will. This same contrast between the philistine and the intellectual person in matters of general human interest also appears, within narrower domains, between the ignorant and the educated, the inexperienced and the experienced, specialists and laypersons, pupils and teachers.

The philistine is unable to discern, within the present, the traces of the past and the germs of the future. He cannot see how the present may serve both to reconstruct what has been and to anticipate what is to come. He fails to distinguish between accidental, imagined, subjective, and merely apparent relations on the one hand, and essential, permanent, causal, and real relations on the other. He also confuses spiritual possessions with material ones. Compared with the slow, hesitant, groping inferences of the philistine and even of the talented individual, the conclusions of the genius give the impression of intuition. Where the talented person reasons, the genius perceives. Where the talented person searches without finding, the genius finds without searching. Where the talented person sees obscurity and confusion, the genius perceives clarity and obvious relations.

Thinking, or reason, never transcends experience. By reasoning we do not obtain more than what experience—perception and feeling—has already given us. Reason can only analyze and synthesize the data of experience; it cannot increase their quantity. When we infer the future from the present, it is because experience has taught us that the future stands to the present as the present stands to the past: what is prominent today was once only a tendency, and what appears tentative now may become reality tomorrow. When we infer a whole class from a few known instances, it is because experience shows that things or events sharing one property often share others as well. Experience teaches us not only what is, but also what ought to be; for the "ought" is itself one of the actual tendencies of reality. The ideal is an exceptional or embryonic reality; the future exists in germ within the present.

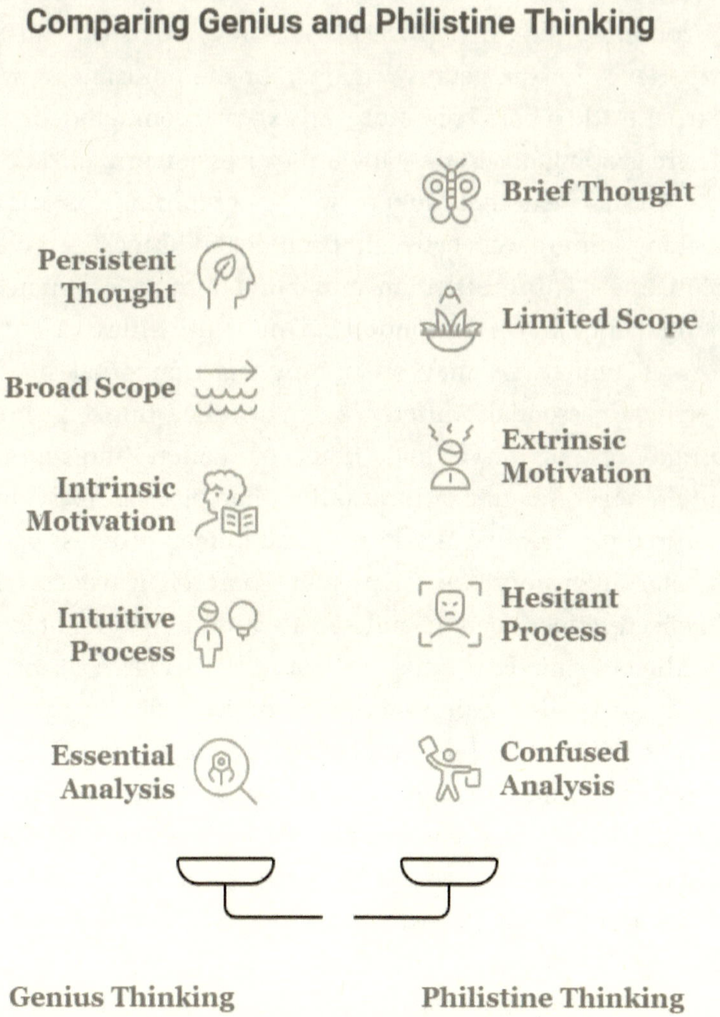

If genius appears to transcend experience, it is because the experience of the genius is richer and more consciously aware of both origin and direction than that of the talented person or the philistine. The mental eye of the genius is attuned to perceive tendencies and nascent movements, while others are absorbed by loud and obvious facts. He seeks deep similarities and inner unity, whereas others remain captivated by superficial diversity. What is a clear perception, a conscious inner command, a purposeful striving (Zweckbewusstes Streben), an actual experience for the genius remains, for the philistine, a dream, a partial truth, a bold conjecture, an external command, or a vague desire groping uncertainly toward expression or realization.

Formal, external, superficial, geographical, historical, and striking differences between people and things captivate the philistine's entire attention and blind him to essential, inner, permanent, and time-independent similarities. Conversely, formal similarities may so occupy his mind that he fails to perceive essential differences. For the thinker, however, differences of place and time, of nation and epoch, are differences of degree or form rather than of essence. Evolution is not so much creative as selective, and human progress lies less in greater intensity than in greater comprehensiveness. Higher intellect, refined feeling, and elevated morality are not exclusive products of modern times or of any particular race; they have always existed, but find increasing opportunity and acceptance. Just as railways and telegraphs have reduced physical distances between human beings, so insight into the permanent similarities beneath changing forms reduces the psychological distance between them. Where the philistine perceives only chaos and discord, deeper vision reveals underlying order and a growing harmony.

All mental processes, even the simplest and most fleeting, pass through stages of growth and decline. A sensation, when attended to, begins as a vague, undifferentiated experience lacking clear quality or location. Gradually it becomes more definite, acquiring recognizable intensity, duration, and localization. Under favorable conditions, such a sensation may develop into perception, apperception—that is, perception combined with memory—conception, and finally a general view. An incipient perception or recollection begins as something vague and unnameable; only if attention is sustained does it become clearer, more differentiated, and properly classified as new or familiar, local or contextual.

The same holds for concepts. The idea of a class of things or of a common property often begins as a dim suspicion that only after days, months, or even years—if ever—takes on a clearly defined form. The dissolution of a mental process reverses this course. When, after arriving at a clear decision regarding what to do and how, where, and why to do it, attention is suddenly diverted by a vivid perception or memory, the decision may sink back into the subconscious. At first we remember only that a decision was made, but not how or why; later we may recall nothing except the vague sense that something had once been resolved.

Let us now return to our central theme—the contrast between superior and average minds—and apply to it the psychological principles outlined above. In the philistine mind, mental processes, especially conceptual ones, rarely advance beyond an embryonic stage marked by vagueness, indefiniteness, and lack of clear individual character. Unbalanced, nebulous, immature, decaying, or mystical thinkers may at times raise their conceptions close to the level of clarity and intellectual security; yet either their courage or their strength fails. They grow dizzy at the height and allow their concepts to slip back into the dark depths of unconsciousness, confusion, and uncertainty. Only the balanced intellectual genius succeeds in sustaining certain ideas at the luminous heights of clear and stable thought. Likewise, only the ideal person of action—the volitional genius—is fully conscious of his wishes, aspirations, and the means of realizing them.

The volitional philistine knows only that he wishes to live differently, without having the faintest notion of what this difference entails. Volitional talent may know what it longs for, yet it lacks the knowledge of how to translate desire into reality. The emotionally talented individual feels a powerful pressure of feeling within the heart; but how to release this feeling, how to bring this emotional germ into the light of day, to nurture it to maturity and social usefulness—this task belongs to the emotional genius.

The normal average person is intellectually anthropocentric and emotionally egocentric, which is not identical with egoism. The intellectually superior individual is intellectually cosmocentric and emotionally ego- or anthropocentric. The morally superior person is both intellectually and emotionally anthropocentric.

The common individual turns to disinterested thinking only when free from material anxieties; the superior individual does so despite the cares and troubles of daily life. The thinking function of the common person—especially of women—has not yet become fully differentiated. It possesses no independent energy of its own and operates only when there is a surplus of vitality or under the pressure of immediate necessity. It is intermittent, accidental, and unstable. Common sense reasons sanely, but rarely with clarity; philosophical speculation, by contrast, reasons clearly, though not always sanely.

The moral philistine, once he has secured a patch of solid ground amid the stormy sea of life, may begin to take interest in the fate of his less fortunate fellows who are tossed about by merciless waves. He may then come to regard concern for others not merely as eccentricity. The moral genius, however, is profoundly pained by the sight of his fellow human beings drowning. He devises plans to bring them to the firm ground that he sees extending nearby in abundance, even while he himself struggles amid unstable, raging waves and risks being swallowed by the abyss at any moment.

The artistic philistine becomes aware of nature's beauty only after he has been freed from material anxieties and economic insecurity. Nature, with her elemental and untamed forces—the ocean with its furious waves—is beautiful to contemplate but terrible to confront. Just as one cannot delight in the strength of wild beasts before they are rendered harmless, so nature could not be admired before her forces were understood and tamed. Until geniuses taught humanity how to domesticate natural forces, animals, and plants, how to prepare for the future, nature was—and for many still remains—a reservoir of hostile powers and lurking dangers. Her beauties were unnoticed by primitive people whose entire energy was consumed by the struggle for survival.

As civilization advances and understanding grows, nature's terrors recede. With increasing knowledge, compliance with natural laws, and mastery over natural forces, humanity gains ever firmer ground from which to contemplate safely the remaining untamed domains. The genius, for whom ideals are not mere dreams but anticipated future realities, whose mental vision perceives potentialities as near-actualities, can enjoy the beauty of nature in anticipation, even while she still treats him harshly. The moral genius can rejoice in advance over the possibilities of a future humane society, even while suffering under the injustices of the present, because he sees the future embryonically contained in the now and is content with minimal material gratification in order to devote his energy to higher aims.

Mental Harmony

In the mind of the average individual there appears to be harmony between the most contradictory states of consciousness, much as there seems to be harmony among isolated savage groups that never encounter one another. This condition is neither true harmony nor disharmony; it is anharmony. Genuine harmony presupposes conflict. The harmony of the superior mind resembles that of civilized nations that have learned the value of cooperation through the bitter experience of war.

The majority of average people live amid constant contradictions between words and deeds, opinions and behavior. These inconsistencies arise because they lack self-scrutiny and because their beliefs are imposed from without rather than formed through inner development. Their contradictions exist more for observers than for themselves. The average individual is not illogical; he is alogical. His mind is not disharmonious but an-harmonious—fragmented into disconnected compartments. True mental disharmony belongs chiefly to the thinking person, either at the beginning or at the decline of intellectual evolution.

In the average mind, cruelty and kindness, superstition and sound judgment, predatory and cooperative impulses coexist without conflict because there is no unifying, self-examining higher organ to bring them into relation. Emotions possess a diffusive and directly communicative character, whereas ideas and convictions are concentrative and only indirectly communicative. Hence, contradictory emotions cannot coexist simultaneously; they neutralize one another or alternate. Even philistines may achieve emotional harmony, despite contradictions among their beliefs. Harmony among ideas and convictions is established indirectly through their emotional accompaniments. Only beliefs that arise from within—from the depths of the self—are rooted in strong emotion. When a new theory is presented to an original thinker who already holds views on the subject, he immediately feels whether it accords with his own ideas, even before he can articulate logical arguments. He senses agreement or opposition through the emotional resonance of the ideas themselves.

By contrast, the convictions of the philistine and of the semi- or pseudo-superior individual, being imposed from without, remain superficial and emotionally rootless.

They are grafted onto selfish motives and desires, and thus lack inner coherence. This explains why such individuals can assent simultaneously to contradictory doctrines—to religion and science, knowledge and superstition, capitalism and socialism. Their sole test of a new theory is not its truth, but whether it serves personal advantage, avoids offending influential figures, or enhances popularity.

Difference in Affection and Volition

In the evolution of mental life from the average individual to the thinker, a consistent law governs the affective and volitional spheres. What the thinker gains in duration and clarity, he loses in rapidity and intensity. Irritability, impulsiveness, and intolerance gradually give way to sensibility, deliberation, and tolerance. In psychology, as in mechanics, the products duration × rapidity and clarity × intensity remain essentially constant as we move from the unthinking to the thinking stage.

The affections of the philistine—especially of women—show characteristic traits.

(a) They are intense and quickly aroused, but inconstant, short-lived, and vague, often unconscious of their origin and aim.

(b) There is little differentiation or purity of feeling. Sentiments lack independence: the object of love becomes simultaneously an object of admiration, sexual attraction, pride, hope, joy, envy; the object of hatred is also an object of contempt, anger, fear, shame, and sorrow. Self-love is inseparably mixed with vanity. Thus poverty and the poor become at once objects of pity, contempt, ridicule, antipathy, and dread, while wealth and the wealthy evoke desire, worship, admiration, affection, and confidence.

(c) There is an excessive extension or transfer of feeling from one quality of an object to all its other qualities—even those that would, in themselves, provoke the opposite sentiment. The philistine cannot admire a person's intelligence while despising his character; he cannot love merits and also recognize defects.

(d) Feelings are unduly transferred to objects only superficially or accidentally connected with the original object of love or hate. Love or hatred for a person, nation, or race extends to possessions, clothing, pets, manners, language, and customs.

(e) Affections are often evoked by mere form, symbol, name, or outwardly insignificant features—visible in fetishism, idolatry, superstition, and collective antipathies.

(f) Between opposite emotions there are few or only embryonic intermediate states. Especially in women, feelings may swing abruptly from love to hatred without passing through sympathy, politeness, indifference, or antipathy; from enthusiasm and confidence to distrust and despair without intermediate stages.

(g) The philistine mistakes interested, associative, heteronomous feeling for disinterested, autonomous affection.

(h) He is philoneistic—seeking novelty—in sensations and emotions, but misoneistic—averse to novelty—in ideas. The opposite holds for the scientific and philosophical genius. Artists and poets find new emotional depths in old objects; the philistine seeks new emotions by changing objects. This partly explains the rapid spread of intoxicants, fashions, and novelties, and why modern people differ from earlier generations more in objects of affection than in the affections themselves.

(i) Alongside confused thinking runs confused feeling. Narrow judgments correspond to narrow sympathies, misplaced affections, undeserved antipathies, and emotional excess at the wrong time and in wrong proportion. Most opinions and most affections of the philistine are imposed from without through hetero-suggestion.

Adaptation, Heredity, and Variability

Adaptation

The genius anticipates the future. The common individual adapts to present circumstances; the genius adapts to ideal future conditions potentially contained in the present. Like a converging lens, the genius gathers the weak, unconscious, scattered tendencies of the masses into a luminous, conscious, life-producing focus. The direct influence of the social and cosmic environment rarely reaches consciousness in the average mind; it enters only through the suggestive mediation of the genius, and often in mutilated form.

Left to himself, the common individual adapts negatively—by flight, forgetting, renunciation; by drowning thought in restless activity; by indulgence in illusion, stupefaction, intoxicants; by retreat into torpor, sleep, ecstasy, or mysticism. The genius produces positive adaptation—by changing the environment, the self, or both. The sane genius is highly adaptable: his mental equilibrium is stable, and environmental influences shift his center of interest gradually and proportionately. The insane person has unstable equilibrium: a trivial cause may suddenly overthrow his vital center. The average individual adapts only under the joint influence of circumstances and geniuses; his equilibrium is indifferent, and without guidance he cannot shift his inner balance appropriately.

The male is variable, adaptable, teachable, acquisitive, and original; the female is stable, conservative, imitative, and individually unprogressive. Many men born into privilege adapt, when compelled, to harsh and uncertain lives; women born in poverty rarely adapt to deprivation when luxuries are withdrawn. Easy ascent into higher ranks does not prove adaptability; smooth paths demand little effort, and aristocratic conventions are familiar to imitation and display.

Intelligence primarily means the ability to adapt to changing and uncertain conditions with minimal action, minimal energy, and minimal loss. Animal and philistine adaptation consists in flight or blind persistence. Human and original adaptation neither flees into torpor nor exhausts itself in harmful activity; it seeks the most economical transformation of self or environment. The genius—and humanity, unlike animals—is not overactive or inert; he avoids useless muscular effort. The moral genius appears less adapted to current society than the amoral or immoral, who have nothing to guard. The genuine intellectual genius, for whom thinking is an end in itself, seems less adapted than the pseudo-superior, for whom thinking is a means to comfort; yet he saves energy by renouncing vanity and luxury.

The moral genius does not wage war on human aversion to muscular effort; he knows progress lies in brain development, not muscle. He condemns laziness that exploits others, and honors reflective mastery of natural forces. He detests both drudgery and torpor—both waste life.

Lower bodily adaptation is passive and submissive, seen in plants and cold-blooded animals whose life fluctuates with environment and may suspend under extremes. Primitive adaptation to food scarcity includes gorging when abundant and starvation when scarce—internal sacrifice to preserve essentials. Higher adaptation actively reduces dependence on fluctuation: warm-blooded regulation, food storage, and agriculture.

What holds for bodily adaptation applies also to psychic and social adaptation. A lower, philistine social adaptation allows convictions and feelings to shift with surroundings. The adult philistine becomes increasingly imitative and suggestible—believing with believers, doubting with skeptics, cynical with cynics, tyrannical with exploiters—or he abandons thinking altogether, becoming docile, inert, and indifferent.

The higher form of adaptation to the social environment is that of the genius, who either shapes for himself a social world in harmony with his own convictions and sentiments, or consciously maintains a certain distance from others in order to protect his individuality from the oppressive weight of imposed beliefs. Unlike the emotionally driven individual, whose inner balance is easily disturbed by the changing fortunes of life and the capricious fluctuations of human affection, the intellectually developed individual is equipped with effective inner safeguards.

These psychical self-protective mechanisms enable him to preserve mental equilibrium and stability. He clearly distinguishes reality from appearance, realizable wishes from unrealizable ones. He eliminates vanity and illusory ambitions—desires whose fulfillment depends entirely upon the favor or will of others. He transforms dreams into workable realities, avoids excessive intimacy with unstable and capricious individuals, and learns to regulate and calm emotional upheavals when they arise. By these means he maintains an inner climate of clarity, balance, and independence, even amid the pressures and fluctuations of social life. The more rapidly a living being develops in a particular direction or along a specific evolutionary path, and the farther it advances along that path, the less capable it becomes of changing direction and following a new and higher course. The more an organism is molded by its environment, the less capable it is of molding, transforming, or improving that environment. The more perfectly an animal is adapted to a given environment, the less adaptable it proves when that environment changes.

The philistine and the individual belonging to an inferior race are bodily more developed—that is, closer to the mature simian type—than the intellectual individual and the person belonging to a superior race, who bodily remain nearer to the infantile type. What is gained in adaptation to a fixed environment is lost in adaptability to a new one. The more narrowly we confine ourselves to a few immediate aims, the less capable we become of pursuing broader, more distant, or still unrealized ends.

In order to live, one must be adapted in some degree to one's surroundings. The degenerate individual is unadaptable, though not unadapted. More precisely, he is actively but not passively unadaptable. He survives only because he has found simple, frictionless conditions, but he would perish if these conditions were altered or removed. An extreme form of degeneration would be to be both actively and passively unadaptable—incapable of surviving any change in habitual life.

The actively adaptable individual is dissatisfied with existing conditions and capable of initiating change. He resists, selects, modifies, and subdues external influences, asserting and reshaping his inborn tendencies. The merely adapted individual is passively adjustable to slow change but incapable of responding to rapid or sudden transformations. He is imitative, submissive, yielding, self-renouncing, and highly suggestible.

In prehistoric times, bodily stronger but psychically less adaptable dark races displaced the bodily weaker yet psychically more adaptable white race from the warm zones, which demanded little initiative or exertion from their inhabitants.

Heredity

Heredity signifies the persistence and transmission of past environmental influences—that is, of the organism's reactions to them—as long as the provoking conditions remain unchanged or vary only slightly. The genius inherits from his parents a tendency to react in modified ways to environmental change. The philistine inherits more primitive, fixed, and organized modes of reaction. The genius inherits the potential, undeveloped, socially unprotected, variable mental tendencies of his ancestors, whereas the philistine inherits their developed, localized, secure, socially approved mental possessions.

What was in the ancestors only a tentative, secondary mode of reaction becomes in the genius a natural, primary one. Conversely, the ancestors' primary reactions—struggle for food, shelter, rank, reproduction—become secondary in the genius, subordinated to intellectual, social, or moral ideals. He is prepared to reduce them to a minimum or sacrifice them when they conflict with higher aims.

Experiences acquired during an individual's lifetime cannot destroy natural impulses nor create new ones; they can only slightly modify inherited tendencies. A person naturally devoted to truth cannot become a successful habitual deceiver, regardless of painful experiences caused by honesty. Yet experiences accumulate across generations as instincts and emotions, provided environmental conditions remain similar. The more intellectually gifted an individual is, the more easily he frees himself from inherited impulses that no longer fit his environment, or reshapes his environment to support his natural inclinations. Fear of darkness or animals was once a necessary inheritance for prehistoric humans living amid constant danger.

In a modern individual, such phobias—unsupported by experience—represent degeneration, atavism, or philistine inertia. Likewise, instinctive cruelty or suspicion toward strangers, once justified in hostile tribal environments, becomes pathological or reactionary conservatism in a civilized society that demands altruism and openness.

Variability and Progress

Progress, evolution, and development signify adaptive change—change that benefits the organism. Progress does not imply constant, rapid, or chaotic variation. It means change at the right moment and in the right direction.

Language, for example, progresses not through rapid variation but through increasing clarity, economy, and stability. Progress does not necessarily mean novelty or complexity; it may require a return to simpler, older forms. It is defined more by its aims and results than by its means, more by content than by form. Progress rarely occurs uniformly across all functions of an individual or society. It may require temporary stagnation or regression in some areas. Both the genius and the philistine exhibit variability, but in the philistine it is weak and unorganized. He lacks the intelligence to select adaptive variations and eliminate maladaptive ones. His variability remains latent until stimulated by geniuses whose variability is irrepressible. Thus the philistine is variable but not progressive—imitative rather than creative, original in trivial form but not in meaningful content. What constitutes progress for an individual or a class may represent regression for humanity as a whole; what benefits humanity may be irrelevant to the universe. What is disadvantageous for the genius may yield benefits for society. From the social standpoint, the genius is more adaptable than the philistine, though from the narrow standpoint of personal survival the philistine often appears better fitted. This apparent advantage arises from imitation and surface adjustment, not from genuine understanding of progress.

Women often seem more adaptable than men because they are rarely placed in truly novel circumstances. Across times and societies they are assigned essentially the same role, though expressed in different languages and costumes. The role remains constant; only its outward forms change.

Progress means moving ever closer to one's aims and goals. Human progress, or civilization, signifies a qualitative and quantitative increase in the realization of economic, intellectual, emotional, aesthetic, and moral ends. It involves greater security of livelihood, an expanding range of means for satisfying bodily needs, increased certainty and breadth of knowledge, a richer variety of sources for healthy enjoyment, and a growth in happiness, solidarity, love, liberty, and respect for individuality among human beings. In short, progress enriches and intensifies human life; it lengthens life spiritually, if not materially, and increases it in quality, even when it cannot increase it in quantity. Herbert Spencer's formula of evolution, when applied to human societies, emphasizes formal and external aspects but fails to grasp the inner core, the living soul of progress. As a daring attempt to survey an immense and complex field from the heights of philosophical generalization, Spencer's effort deserves admiration. Yet admiration for the boldness of the undertaking must not blind us to the meagerness of the results achieved. The means by which progress is realized is active adaptation: the transformation of cosmic and social environments; the creation of safer, more stable, and more favorable artificial conditions; the domestication of physical and psychological forces; the elimination of harmful variations in both self and environment; and the recognition and cultivation of useful variations.

Difference in Racial Influence

Bodily differences among races are more pronounced and more natural than psychological differences. Geniuses belonging to different races differ even less psychologically than average individuals of different races. This becomes clear when we remember that the body adapts to relatively stable physical conditions limited in time and space, whereas the mind is both a product and a factor of superior adaptation to unstable, changing physical and social circumstances—past, present, and possible. Races inhabit different geographic environments, but intellectually they live, or tend to live, in the same world. While actual circumstances vary, possible circumstances are common to all humanity. Hence the striking uniformity of philosophical temperament across the globe.

Externally and bodily, human beings are shaped by and dependent upon their physical and social surroundings. Mentally, however, the superior individual masters and reshapes the environment in accordance with inner needs and aspirations, achieving a relative independence from it. The richer and stronger one's inner mental life—that is, the greater one's genius—the less one is bound by physical and social circumstances, and the less one is influenced by so-called racial or national mental traits. These traits are not permanent or natural, as some ethnological psychologists claim, but superficial, changeable, artificial, and often the result of philistine imitation enforced by socially dominant pseudo-superior figures.

Genius and Nationality

The more isolated a community, tribe, or nation, the less freedom, solitude, and independence its individual members enjoy, and the fewer the thought-stimulating influences acting upon them. As intercourse among nations increases, individual originality and healthy peculiarity grow, while rigid national traits diminish. National and individual originality are inversely related. What appears as national peculiarity is largely uniformity among individuals—an enforced one-sidedness of development.

Differences between nations do not consist in fundamental psychological contrasts, but in the emphasis or greater frequency of certain universally human qualities in some groups and of other qualities in others. That such national traits are superficial and artificial is demonstrated by the fact that children of immigrants do not differ psychologically from native-born children. The offspring of supposedly impulsive and emotional Italians may grow into reserved, calculating, intellectually oriented Americans; a child born of a people reputed to be peace-loving and monotheistic may be raised to become militant, fanatical, or polytheistic.

The more original an individual is, the fewer national characteristics he exhibits. Geniuses of different nationalities resemble one another physically and psychologically far more than they resemble their own countrymen. Even average individuals of different nations but of the same profession often resemble and understand one another more readily than compatriots of different occupations. The division of humanity into nations is largely artificial and accidental. Patriotism frequently disguises class interests: rulers and capitalists of different nations intermarry freely, yet consider it degrading to marry someone of a lower social or economic class from their own nation.

Attitude Toward the Established Order

The average person accepts the world and its institutions as a fixed, indisputable reality. The superior individual of extreme moral idealism denies the existing order any justification for existence. The balanced idealist, however, regards the world and society as a complex of facts in the process of transformation—capable of being reshaped and improved.

In the average mind, desire, belief, and knowledge are not clearly differentiated processes—still less so in women. One neither believes nor seeks to know what one does not wish to be true. Convictions of superiority, immortality, or destiny are held because they are desired. The thinking individual, by contrast, seeks to know reality in order to modify desires and beliefs accordingly, whenever possible. When the average person becomes sentimental, he oscillates between hope and fear, between naïve optimism and despairing pessimism. The balanced superior mind adheres to meliorism—a sober confidence in gradual improvement.

Modern pragmatism represents a regression to this undifferentiated, philistine mode of thought. William James, one of the most brilliant modern sophists, openly dethrones logic. In The Will to Believe, he reduces truth to a product of belief; in Pragmatism and The Meaning of Truth, he takes a further step backward by subordinating both knowledge and belief to utility and desire.

For the average person, the ideal exists either somewhere already realized or nowhere at all. For the superior individual, the ideal is projected into the future. Ideals of perfection, justice, and goodness are conceived by the inferior mind as actual, external realities—Gods or paradises existing in distant realms. The superior mind conceives them as internal and potential possibilities, toward which humanity gradually approaches—like a curve approaching its asymptote—tending toward realization over infinite time.

Men of genius stand at the periphery of the human phalanx. They are in closer contact with the surrounding environment, with the cosmic and social milieu. They receive the first shocks, the earliest impacts, which they transmit in a mitigated form to the great mass of humanity. At the same time, they gather the unconscious reactions of the masses and transform them into conscious, seemingly spontaneous responses directed back toward the environment.

The philistine entertains a blind and disinterested reverence for established institutions and prevailing opinions. He judges their soundness by the number of adherents, without regard to the psychological or moral differences among those adherents. To him, institutions appear indisputable, immutable, almost divine—beyond understanding and beyond criticism. The pseudo-superior individual, by contrast, is an interested and insincere worshiper of success. He never attacks a harmful social institution or an erroneous system of beliefs as long as it remains powerful and popular, as long as it is profitable to remain on good terms with it. Nor does he defend a nascent theory or a newly forming institution while doing so entails danger, risk, or lack of reward.

Only the genuine genius refuses to be swept along by the current of blind or interested worship, by imposing externals, by the weight of tradition, or by the halo of the past. For him, the sole justification of theories, beliefs, and opinions lies in their degree of truth. The only claim to existence that social organs or institutions possess is their social usefulness—that is, their ability to perform more effectively and more economically functions that individuals or private groups can fulfill only imperfectly. Just as in the individual organism cutaneous respiration does not render pulmonary breathing superfluous, and cutaneous elimination does not replace the kidneys, so social institutions justify their privileged position only by their indispensable service to the whole.

The philistine's conservatism—his reverence for and idealization of the existing order—is merely the reverse side of his aversion to deep, far-reaching change. Thus, the proletarian philistine may recognize the usefulness of trade unions in forcing higher wages or improved working conditions, yet he cannot advance further with socialists or industrial unionists toward the abolition of exploitation itself. Similarly, aristocratic or predatory philistines may concede a few superficial reforms; but even when they proclaim themselves liberals or progressives, they remain committed to preserving a social order founded upon overt or disguised oppression and exploitation of the weak, the poor, the defenseless, and the foreign—condemning them to precarious livelihoods or lifelong drudgery.

True and False Superiority

The truly superior individual—superior by vocation and inner calling—strives to become better and wiser than he is. The sensational, self-advertising, professional pseudo-superior strives merely to appear superior to others. These two tendencies—the will to be superior and the will to be recognized as superior—exclude one another. Hence the delayed, often posthumous but enduring recognition of genuine idealists, and the rapid, noisy, yet fleeting fame of heroes of the day, as perishable as the crowds that applaud them.

The pedant, the financial aristocrat, and the intellectually pseudo-superior individual are far more eager than the genuine scholar to impress others with their supposed superiority through refined language, manners, appearances, company, and surroundings.

The liar and the hypocrite feel a stronger need than the sincere person to emphasize their honesty, to embellish their motives, and to surround themselves with favorable appearances—precisely because they themselves lack inner conviction. The pseudo-superior individual believes in his own excellence only insofar as he succeeds in making others believe in it.

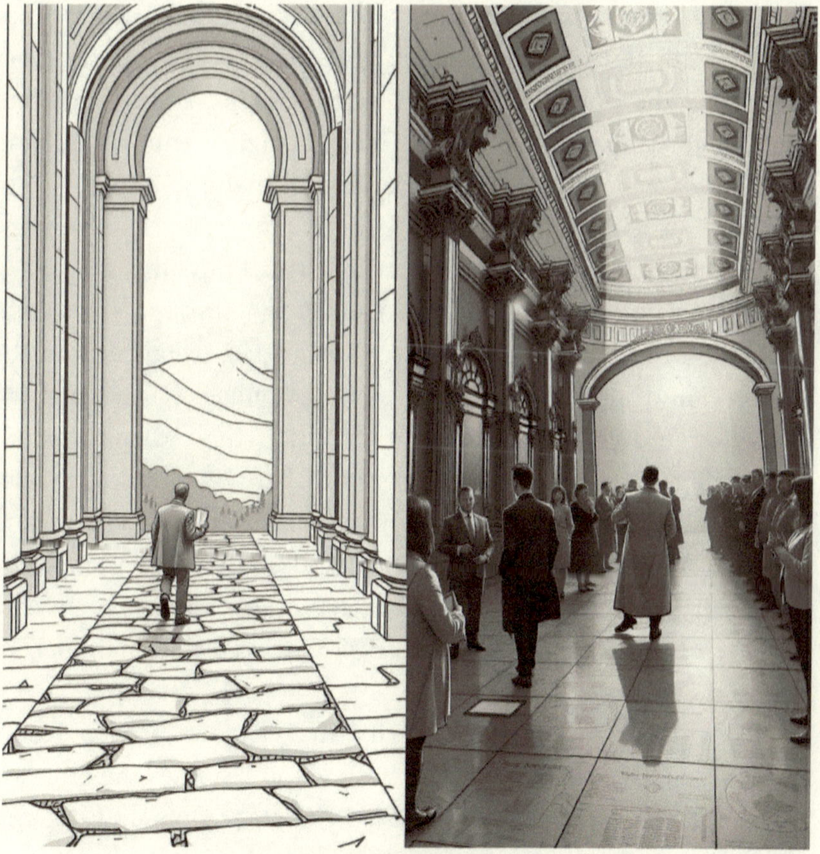

The knowledge of the pseudo-superior individual is superficial and verbal, casually gathered from lectures, conversations, journalistic accounts, and second-hand criticisms. The ideas of the genuinely superior mind are painstakingly formed through personal experience and observation, or patiently drawn from direct engagement with the original works of sincere thinkers. The pseudo-superior learns just enough to conceal ignorance and to give the illusion of deeper understanding.

Pseudo-superior individuals appear many-sided, but their ideas lack inner connection, and their opinions lack harmony with their actions. They do not approach the world from inner necessity or evolutionary impulse; they are guided by fashion and social prestige rather than by inner conviction. Their pursuit is not truth but notoriety, fame, and success. They differ from average individuals less in their inner thinking and feeling than in outward expression—in refined slang, mannerisms, and public demeanor. Their distinction is external and apparent, not internal and real; verbal knowledge replaces genuine understanding, and ostentation masks trivial pursuits.

They cultivate intellectual snobbery through rare and inflated words, theatrical gestures, cultivated distance from the masses, and an atmosphere of assumed mystery. The genuine superior individual does not squander time displaying or exploiting his superiority. He seeks to be, not to seem, greater than he is. The pseudo-superior gratifies personal vanity and selfish ambition, advertising himself indirectly while pretending to glorify a profession, class, sect, nation, or race. His egotism hides beneath the cloak of professional, sectarian, national, or racial megalomania.

For the pseudo-superior individual, truth is accepted only insofar as it serves personal interest; value becomes the criterion of truth. The ideal individual, by contrast, accepts and defends truth even when it conflicts with personal advantage. Only in ethical matters—where human will plays a role—does he test truth by social value. To the pseudo-superior, ethical, religious, artistic, philosophical ideas are ceremonial garments, donned on public occasions and displayed on platforms, in classrooms, or in books—but not worn in everyday life, nor made the guiding substance of action.

The pseudo-superior individual does not love knowledge, truth, art, or religion for their own sake, nor for their universal human value. He values them only insofar as they yield material advantage. He treats them as private property—something to be guarded, monopolized, and exploited as a source of power over those who lack it, over laymen and the ignorant. Thus, he carries the egoistic habits of the economic world into the intellectual and spiritual realms, as far as the spirit of the age permits.

Modern Western pseudo-superior groups no longer form openly sealed castes like the ancient priesthoods or the Brahmins of old. Yet the attentive observer can still detect remnants of caste spirit—caste secrecy, caste arrogance, and an interested solidarity euphemistically called esprit de corps—among academicians, politicians, and members of the so-called liberal professions. Worse still, one often discovers among them a predatory or gang-like spirit. Despite persistent efforts to monopolize knowledge, art, and religion, along with their material rewards, the intellectual world is increasingly permeated by an international, socialistic, and hospitable spirit, preparing the ground for broader social cooperation and, eventually, for community of material goods in the economic sphere.

The genuine superior individual is too rich in original thought and too independent of fleeting public applause to resort to the intellectual dishonesty practiced by pseudo-superiors: obscure and dazzling language, mystical vagueness, deliberately puzzling theories, distortion of simple truths, plagiarism, or the feeding of audiences with empty words and fashionable nonsense. He has no need to intoxicate others with verbal brilliance or theoretical fog.

The genuine superior person adopts the intellectual and moral world as a permanent dwelling place, much as the independent pioneer ventures into new lands to build a lasting home for himself and others. The intellectual realm is not a natural habitat for the semi-superior, and still less for the pseudo-superior individual. At most, such people venture into it briefly, seeking sensational discoveries to report back to the sedentary, conservative masses, who—though resistant to real change—delight in hearing about marvelous possibilities from afar. The semi-superior individual in the intellectual world resembles the predatory pioneer or adventurous traveler who explores unknown regions not in order to live there, but to satisfy curiosity, to impress others, and to earn fame, money, or prestige. Pseudo-superior academicians and professional moralists occupy, in the realm of ideas, the same position that politicians, demagogues, and office-seekers occupy in practical life. They pose as originators of new intellectual movements while doing everything possible to suppress, discourage, or silence genuine contemporary thinkers whose rivalry they fear. Likewise, volitional pseudo-superiors present themselves as social reformers and benefactors, while persecuting or destroying authentic reformers whom they sense may one day replace them as public awareness grows.

The genuine superior individual strives quietly and modestly toward self-perfection—toward surpassing himself rather than others. He is driven by an inner evolutionary impulse, not by envy, ambition, or the compulsion to compete. The noisy competitiveness of semi- and pseudo-superiors is merely a softened form of the primitive fighting instinct, still celebrated in society as a mark of manliness. By contrast, the sincerity, harmlessness, and straightforwardness of genuine superiority point toward the emergence of a cooperative instinct. What is now only a rational demand for collaboration will, in a more advanced society, become an emotional and instinctive one, replacing aggressiveness and servile obedience.

In all their actions, pseudo-superior individuals assume an air of grave importance, creating the illusion that they take their work seriously and regard it as the central purpose of their lives. Only the discerning observer recognizes the actor behind the mask and perceives that self-aggrandizement is the true aim.

Like an actor, the pseudo-superior may at times deceive himself, momentarily identifying with the noble role he performs.

In the intellectual sphere, pseudo-superiors treat knowledge much as financial aristocrats and certain social groups treat people. They zealously maintain artificial boundaries between disciplines, concern themselves more with method and terminology than with truth, and value style, form, and exposition above ideas themselves. They care more about the author of an idea and its usefulness to their own interests than about its truth or relevance to humanity. Formal, abstract, verbal logic is preferred over concrete, living reasoning. Their works, when they produce any, display elegance, fashionable methods, excessive systematization, hypnotic language, mathematical trappings, and an air of mystery—but lack genuine, socially valuable insight.

Like children and women, the pseudo-superior individual strives for authority, power, social distinction, and linguistic wealth—mere symbols of superiority. He imagines that possession of the symbol will automatically bring the reality it represents, or hopes that others will mistake appearance for essence. The craving for power and sham superiority is a remnant of primitive predatory instincts inherited from aggressive nomadic groups that once dominated peaceful agricultural peoples. The instinctive respect or fear shown by the masses toward such sham superiors—even when they lack real power—is a relic of ancient terror before despotic rulers and conquering invaders.

Because the pseudo-superior seeks power and distinction rather than truth, he looks for truth—or pretends to look for it—everywhere except where it actually lies. Preferably, he searches in distant lands, among primitive peoples, or in a remote and inaccessible past. He favors complex, abstract, mathematical, or dialectical methods that are incomprehensible and uncontrollable by the majority. He appears to search the heavens for what lies plainly on earth. He chooses obscure, roundabout paths where no one can follow him closely, where he can remain idle while being celebrated as a pioneer expected to return with revelations of imagined new horizons.

The proletarian philistine is openly materialistic and prosaic, openly narrow-minded and narrow-hearted. Yet beneath his rough exterior he often conceals a tender soul, and beneath his crude manners—whether assumed or imposed—there may lie higher aspirations.

The aristocratic philistine, and especially the pseudo-superior individual, represents a different type: a philistine clothed in the outward appearance of a superior man. He hides hardness of heart behind gentle manners, his prosaic and materialistic nature behind memorized poetic phrases, and his egoism beneath the cloak of altruistic pursuits. His soul is ugly, though his form is pleasing. In essence, he is a trafficker in phrases and appearances, dealing in the outward forms of all that is noble and ideal, imitating and mimicking rather than living them.

The parasitical or pseudo-superior individual, who assumes the external appearance of the genuine superior—and often exaggerates it—does so in order to appropriate the honor and reward that rightly belong to the latter for genuine social service. He recalls those primitive tribesmen who, after the confinement of their wives, lie in bed and imitate the pains of childbirth in order to receive the sympathy and congratulations owed to the women alone. The pseudo-superior leaves to the genius the serious, dangerous, thankless work of pioneering. When the new ground has already been prepared and rendered safe for general occupation—or, figuratively, when new doctrines have been clarified and made immune to attack—he steps in, stirs public opinion, and installs himself as leader or executive authority, harvesting admiration and advantage that properly belong to obscure, forgotten, or posthumously honored geniuses.

Had many of today's rulers been born a century earlier, they would not have called themselves defenders of international peace or friends of oppressed peoples—just as today they resist causes such as unemployment, socialism, or child labor, because these movements are still dangerous, insufficiently established, and demand genuine self-denial and sacrifice. The pseudo-superior wages war under the guise of peace, competes while preaching cooperation, serves himself while pretending to serve others, and commits injustice under the appearance of law and order. When the old military form of conflict becomes inefficient, he proclaims himself a champion of peace while employing the more insidious weapon of capital to crush rivals and enslave others, transferring the spirit of war into industry, commerce, politics, education, and religion. He is an innocent-looking criminal, an intelligent-looking fool, a benevolent-looking egoist, an active-looking idler, a dignified-looking trifler, a brave-looking coward, an honest-looking rogue—a beast of prey in sheep's clothing. His emptiness and ignorance are concealed behind ceremonies, formalities, mystifying conventions, and sonorous words.

Sociability

The philistine is more sociable—though less truly social or altruistic—than the superior individual, because his intellectual and emotional needs are less refined. He has no strong convictions to defend, no imperious aspirations beyond food, shelter, reproduction, amusement, and dress. He lacks the insight to distinguish genuine feeling from simulated sentiment, words of the heart from words of the tongue. He has little longing for subtle and invisible possessions such as friendship, love, or fame, and no understanding of the chastity of the soul;

bodily propriety suffices him. Politeness and friendliness satisfy him better than genuine sympathy.

He has no inner problems to think through, no chains of thought to pursue; solitude is therefore unnecessary to him and even terrifying, for his inner world is barren, and he fears being left alone with his own emptiness.

Thinking has become so unnatural to him that reflection appears as a sign of mental disorder, whereas in the superior individual the opposite—thoughtlessness—would be alarming. Revolutionary ideas, which are natural to a social thinker, appear to the ignorant as moral insanity.

The philistine is more communicative because he lacks the discrimination to decide which of his trivial, repetitive thoughts are worth communicating.

He is unaware that what matters to him may be insignificant to others.

The superior individual, by contrast, selects carefully what may interest or benefit others, and this inner selection itself becomes an obstacle to easy sociability. For the philistine, language is not primarily a vehicle of thought or feeling, but a means of social contact, a discharge for surplus energy. Talking is play, not a serious activity, not a bridge between inner worlds, but an end in itself and a source of immediate pleasure.

All human beings share similar bodily needs, though among financial aristocrats these are refined and multiplied. Intellectual needs, however, differ profoundly among superior individuals. Specialization reaches such an extreme that no two superior minds pursue knowledge in quite the same way.

Some delight in observation and experiment, others in speculation or invention; even within the same field, materials and methods differ so widely that such minds rarely meet in person. They encounter one another chiefly through their works. Solitude, even amid admiration, is the price of mental superiority. The sociability of the philistine arises from a simple love of company. The sociability of the pseudo-superior resembles the helpless attachment of a parasite to its host. His motives are self-interest and vanity; his social success stems from his ability to simulate and dissimulate, from his slight superiority over the masses, from indirect self-advertising, from the absence of strong convictions, and from intellectual dishonesty that permits him to play any role.

The superior individual, by contrast, appears unsociable because he lacks the boldness, naïveté, or theatricality required to impose himself. He may be too considerate, too honest, too self-respecting to feign agreement or to act a part. He is too absorbed in lasting concerns to waste time imitating trivial conventions and empty formulas.

Thinking is an essentially private act. Only its results—thoughts and conclusions—can be shared. The process of thinking itself is incommunicable, for to know how one reaches a conclusion is already to have nearly reached it.

Constant sociability therefore demands the renunciation of thinking, a relapse into superficial enjoyment. The same holds for love: intimate affections are private, and their public exhibition invites envy or ridicule. Excessive social intercourse thus undermines originality, truth-seeking, and even love itself, breeding conventionality, superficiality, and emotional shallowness.

As thoughtful individuals become more numerous and less economically dependent, social life will be transformed. Respect for individuality and naturalness will grow; social intercourse will be tempered by freedom, by intervals of solitude, by the ease of withdrawal and return without formalities.

A healthy human life requires a balanced alternation of work and rest, effort and relaxation, sociability and isolation, public intercourse and privacy.

Difference in Intellectual Needs

Needs, unlike luxuries, demand continual or periodic satisfaction. They cannot be neglected without pain or harm. One never tires of them; they are sought instinctively, not by imitation.

Objects of need are not always different in kind from objects of luxury; often the same object becomes a need or a luxury according to quantity and circumstance. The boundary between the two shifts between individuals and even within the same individual, though within fixed limits that preserve health and happiness.

Intellectual pursuits that are organic necessities for the genius are mere luxuries for the philistine. Conversely, many bodily comforts and vanities that appear indispensable to the philistine are dispensable luxuries to the genius.

The philistine possesses no genuine intellectual needs, or only the most rudimentary ones.

He may display curiosity, but not a true thirst for knowledge, nor any ideal aspiration. In the man of talent, intellectual needs are more developed, yet they lack the depth, persistence, and inner urgency required to assert themselves against adverse circumstances.

External conditions and the social milieu accentuate certain intellectual tendencies and determine their direction, while suppressing many others.

Hence, the intellectual productions of the man of talent are voluntary, methodical, systematic, and carefully planned, rich in erudition yet strikingly poor in genuinely new conclusions.

The pseudo-superior individual often possesses some talent and at times even a spark of genius, but he subordinates his limited and superficial intellectual powers to material gain and personal vanity. In the man of genius, by contrast, both the intensity and the direction of intellectual impulses arise from within. For this reason, his intellectual activity is spontaneous and unmethodical, often poor in erudition, yet rich and daring in its conclusions.

The pursuit of uncertain, risky, and not fully attainable ends demands nearly all of one's energy. It is therefore impossible to pursue two such opposing kinds of ends at once. Whoever is inwardly compelled to pursue truth, knowledge, or social happiness must either possess sufficient material security or reduce bodily needs to a minimum whose satisfaction is reasonably assured. No one can rise into the higher intellectual spheres without a firm and secure economic footing from which to take flight.

Conversely, the great mass of laboring people, as well as insatiable materialists, expend nearly all their energy on food, clothing, shelter, social recognition—deserved or not—petty ambitions, and vain luxuries. Yet even they require a minimal, seemingly solid intellectual refuge, a place to retreat when fatigue overtakes them and when a drowsy conscience reproaches them for their materialism. This minimum they find in dogmatic religion or dogmatic science, which spares them the arduous personal journey into the heights of philosophical reflection on such subtle and vital matters as immortality, the origin and aim of life, and the justification and valuation of human activity. Just as the most world-renouncing philosopher requires a minimal economic foundation, so the philistine and materialist require a minimal dogmatic intellectual foundation.

The aristocratic or parasitic philistine pretends to strive for knowledge and education, while in reality he seeks only their appearance—the mastery of a grandiloquent caste language that serves as a badge of privilege and authority over the proletarian masses. This fact is widely known, though rarely admitted by pseudo-superior individuals: successful lecturers, preachers, and educational leaders who refuse to share knowledge openly in public spaces, preferring exclusive fees, imposing buildings, elaborate ceremonies, and flattery. They know that the mere promise of knowledge would not attract aristocratic philistines, nor persuade them to part with money, their sole object of sincere devotion.

Difference in Originality

Strictly speaking, originality does not distinguish the genius from the philistine if by originality we mean merely any difference from the multitude; in that case the term becomes a tautology. But if originality is understood in its true sense—as initiative, inventiveness, mental variability, and the capacity to go beyond imitation, to do more, better, or differently than one has been taught—then a certain degree of originality must be granted even to the philistine. No two individuals are identical, and philistines, especially aristocratic ones, often enjoy being different from their neighbors, mistaking formal or trivial distinctions for superiority.

The philistine is not opposed to change as such. He readily embraces improvements in material comfort, new pleasures, novel sensations, commercial innovations, and technical progress that yield greater returns. What he resists is the mental effort required by higher, disinterested pursuits; he resists changes that demand inner transformation or compliance with the spirit rather than the mere form of new institutions. He opposes radical, substantial change, but welcomes superficial and convenient novelty. He rejects new ends, but gladly accepts better means for achieving familiar ones.

Thus, the alleged opposition between conservatism and progressivism is in truth an opposition between selfish, parasitic, and narrow pursuits on the one hand, and unselfish, productive, and higher pursuits on the other. The genuinely progressive individual never seeks to discard humanity's valuable past; rather, he strives to preserve whatever has proven truly useful.

The essential difference between philistine and superior originality lies here: philistine originality is quantitative and applies itself to trivial amusements, selfish material needs, and minor deviations that provide temporary advantage. The originality of the genius is qualitative. His intellectual powers are not only greater in degree, but his aims differ in kind—broader, more serious, more comprehensive. His originality is directed toward distant, ultimate, and generally useful ends, toward the creation of new ideals and new aims of life.

The originality of aristocratic philistines invents new amusements but not new machines; new words for old ideas; more attractive but not more wholesome food; more ornate but not more hygienic clothing; new appearances without new realities; luxuries without new means of satisfying genuine needs; charity without altruism; legal subtleties without social justice. Their originality lies in disguising base pursuits, not in adopting nobler ones—in inventing methods of deception, domination, self-advertisement, and self-glorification rather than self-perfection.

From such originality one may learn how to waste surplus energy in games, hunting, athletics, idle speculation, or occult amusements, but not how to transform surplus energy into productive thought or socially useful work—how to unite labor with play, mental elevation with enjoyment, and public service with personal fulfillment. One may learn how to appear a benefactor while remaining an idle parasite, how to invent conventions and ceremonies to conceal ignorance, callousness, and egoism.

The originality of proletarian philistines manifests itself in discovering ways to please exploiters or to extract personal advantage from existing conditions, not in improving those conditions. It finds means of enduring or evading evils, not of eliminating them, and derives consolation from illusions rather than from transformation.

The deceptive and antisocial originality of aristocratic philistines reaches its peak in their spokesmen, the pseudo-superior individuals, who—while serving exploiters—pose as leaders of the people to gain the confidence of the exploited. Alongside verbal and formal originality, the pseudo-superior may possess a spark of genuine talent. Yet he degrades and prostitues the art or science in which he is gifted, diverting it from its social mission and pressing it, under disguise, into the service of power and exploitation. Thus talent becomes an instrument of domination rather than a means of enlightenment and human advancement.

When freedom from material anxiety—food, shelter, clothing—leaves the wealthy philistine with a surplus of energy, he usually dissipates it in pleasure-seeking that gradually ruins both mind and body. Only in rare cases does he turn this surplus toward original activity. Yet even then, his originality differs fundamentally from that of the genuine genius. It does not express itself in the creation of new and socially valuable aims, nor in the enrichment of human ideals, but rather in the superficial embellishment of old pursuits and familiar forms.

The rich philistine is intellectually timid. He lacks the courage to venture onto untrodden ground or to move beyond the external aspects of existing or proposed institutions. He prefers to circle around vital problems, remaining within sight of the crowd, rather than to penetrate into their dark interior, where he might find himself alone. His surplus energy is spent on socially harmful play activities and luxuries—refined delicacies, ever-changing fashions in dress or dwelling, etiquette and conventionalities, flirtation, dilettantism, decoration, eccentricities, fads, and useless verbal inventions—rather than on serious and socially fruitful aims such as the pursuit of genuine knowledge, deepened love, or substantial beauty.

What truly distinguishes the genius from the philistine is not the latter's absolute inability to produce new ideas or interpretations, but his fear of the unknown—his fear of straying too far from the multitude—and his lack of intellectual courage to invite others into new regions of thought that he may dimly glimpse. The mercenary or pseudo-superior individual, by contrast, is not afraid of the unknown, yet he lacks a genuine thirst for knowledge and is too attached to personal comfort to venture far into it. Nor does he wish to illuminate the darkness of the unknown, for fear of exposing the poverty of his own insight and because he prefers to exploit the fear and curiosity of the masses who await his return with supposed revelations.

Both the rich philistine, whose superficial education gives him an appearance of intellectual superiority, and the pseudo-superior individual lack the modesty and the disinterested, impersonal, self-forgetful love of knowledge that characterize the genuine superior mind. They venture far enough into intellectual territory to attract attention, but not so far as to risk being forgotten or losing public applause. They never remain long enough in the realms of thought and meditation to be missed by admiring contemporaries. They also lack the intellectual honesty to recognize how little real knowledge remains once academic verbosity and ornamental pseudo-knowledge are stripped away.

This is not because the field of human inquiry is exhausted or finite, but because under present conditions the teacher often lacks either the ability or the means to guide others along the path of independent inquiry. It was not merely fear of intellectual prostitution that led Spinoza to withdraw from notoriety and to refuse a university chair; it was also his modesty and his conviction that he did not yet know enough to teach others, much less to compress truth into a brief academic course. Likewise with Schopenhauer: it was not vanity that led him to lecture on The World as Will and Representation, but his belief that this work contained, for the time being, the most solid knowledge he could responsibly offer.

By contrast, pseudo-superior individuals—among them the overwhelming majority of professors, academic philosophers, priests, moral leaders, journalists, and statesmen—driven by vanity or greed, undertake to teach what they do not truly know, to enlighten others on matters that remain obscure to themselves, and to lead humanity toward goals they neither clearly understand nor sincerely desire to reach.

The dilettantism of wealthy philistines closely resembles the flirtation of shallow and heartless individuals. They do not take art or science seriously. Unlike genuine superior minds, they fail to concentrate sustained love and attention on a single serious pursuit while maintaining respectful interest in others. Their aim is amusement, vanity, and the killing of boredom. In this way, they degrade art and knowledge just as frivolous flirtation degrades love, which in its true form is a serious force in the preservation and elevation of human life.

Semi-superior individuals take intellectual pursuits more seriously, yet their seriousness is conditional. Like those who value affection only when it confers social prestige, they devote themselves chiefly to fashionable scientific or artistic trends. They resemble merchants who deal in goods not out of personal interest, but because the market demands them. In the same way, the pseudo-superior individual treats knowledge, art, and morality as commodities—produced, packaged, and sold in an often diluted and adulterated form.

What has been said of male aristocratic philistines applies equally to female philistines. In early youth and during the childbearing period, many are absorbed primarily in flirtation, love affairs, and sexual parasitism, with little understanding of the wider world in which they live. Those who are not wholly degenerate do assume some maternal responsibility. In later life, however, when maternal duties have ceased, the incurable parasite attempts to relive youthful frivolity, feeding scandal and disturbing the peace of others. Those who are less crippled by parasitic habits may attempt some moral or social development—cultivating friendships, engaging in social welfare, defending women's rights, or spreading knowledge of hygiene. Yet they generally lack the courage, endurance, and self-denial required for more serious pursuits: scientific investigation, radical social reform, sustained care of the poor and the orphaned, or a principled struggle against the tyranny and moral corruption of fashion, luxury, and ostentatious display.

Thus, wherever surplus energy is not guided by inner necessity and moral courage, it tends to degenerate into ornament, play, and exploitation. Only the genuine superior mind transforms surplus energy into lasting insight, social value, and the quiet but enduring advancement of humanity.

End of the Chapter

Chapter-2.
Origins of Genius: Heredity, Variation, and Environment

This chapter uncovers the deep forces that shape exceptional minds—how heredity, variation, and environment converge to kindle originality. By tracing genius to biological inheritance, social conditions, and surplus mental energy, it reveals why greatness cannot be manufactured, yet can be nurtured, and how societies may either suffocate or cultivate their most transformative spirits.

Origin and Conditions– Heredity and Spontaneous Variation

Heredity and variation are inseparable and complementary aspects of reproduction. Neither is more primitive than the other, nor can one be reduced to a special case of the other. Once the fundamental functions of life—nutrition and reproduction—are given, heredity and variation follow necessarily. Life itself implies perpetual change. Parents are never exactly the same at two successive moments, since both their inner and outer environments are continually shifting. How, then, could a child, born into different circumstances, reproduce all parental traits exactly as they appeared at corresponding periods in the parents' lives?

At the same time, the internal and external environment of the fetus and the child overlaps far more closely with that of the parents than with that of any other individuals. It is therefore natural that the child's variations tend to cluster nearer to the parental average than to that of strangers. Every character or trait may be regarded as composed of three elements: one that is inherited; a second that appears to be a variation but is in reality the activation or liberation of a latent parental trait, or conversely the repression of one that was formerly active; and a third that is genuinely new, arising from acquisition under novel conditions. From the subjective point of view, genius often appears spontaneous, as though created out of nothing. Objectively, however, it can be understood as the result of an accumulation and summation of inherited, unconscious tendencies—of cosmical and social impulses transmitted through generations. If heredity meant nothing more than rigid conservation or mechanical copying; if inheritance were uniparental or merely alternating, then genius would indeed be incompatible with heredity. But heredity transmits tendencies, not finished traits. Tendencies that were counteracted, repressed, or neutralized in ancestors may be released and become active in their descendants. Moreover, inheritance is frequently biparental and blended: similar parental characteristics may add together in the child. Under these conditions, heredity and genius are not opposed.

The child is not a mere replica of his parents. He is the continuation of their tendencies, carrying forward the curve of development, whether in its ascending or descending phase. When a genius has reached the summit of his developmental curve—when no further higher potential remains—the child may well be inferior to the parent, at least by comparison.

Hereditary, inner, physiological influences can ultimately be traced back to cumulative environmental, outer, and social influences. Whatever is inherited must once have been acquired in a remote past under the action of the physical and social environment. Only those acquired characteristics that affect the organism deeply—reaching not only the soma but also the germ plasm—are transmitted.

For the emergence of genius, qualitatively similar parental characteristics must combine in an algebraic manner. A mere geometrical addition tends to produce ordinary individuals or those of moderate talent. The algebraic resultant, however, is unstable, which explains why higher genius so often fails to be directly hereditary. When the angle of attraction between two parental characteristics is maximal—symbolically expressed as zero degrees—the resultant equals their sum. This constitutes creative inheritance. It is a well-attested fact that children conceived in mutual attraction and self-forgetful union, untainted by selfish calculation, often display exceptional bodily and mental vigor. When the resultant equals only one of the parental traits, we observe alternate inheritance. When repulsion is maximal—symbolically expressed as one hundred and eighty degrees—the outcome is degenerative inheritance.

Environment

Every human being is at once a product of the environment and an active factor within it. The genius differs from others chiefly in that he is a more powerful factor. Both the working class and the class of geniuses—the physical and the mental workers, the supporting and the genuinely guiding elements of society—arise from the outer layers of the social organism: from those strata that are more exposed to physical and social influences and frictions, yet not entirely worn down by them; from groups that are less protected, less supported, and less guided.

The immediate environment exerts a less obvious influence on the individual life of the genius than on that of the average person. Its effects are clearer in the life of races and species than in that of individuals, and more pronounced on the mind than on the body. With heredity, the reverse holds true: its influence is more evident in the philistine than in the genius, more evident in the individual than in the race, and more evident in the body than in the mind. Environmental influences accumulate over time, which gives original creations the appearance of spontaneity. In the genius, remote and latent environmental forces are concentrated into an intense, active focus. Within individual life, the object upon which tendencies act appears more environmentally determined than their magnitude and direction, which are largely inborn.

In theory, the environment of a being comprises everything in the universe except itself. In practice, it includes only those things and beings that can actually act upon it. Human beings, especially in their social relations, select much of their environment. This makes it difficult to disentangle external influences from personal abilities, compulsion from choice, and suggestion from originality. Strong individuality and pronounced originality lead one to avoid associations in which one cannot express or even preserve one's nature. Throughout history, superior women—such as the cultivated companions of ancient Athens—have sought select circles or withdrawn into convents, salons, or literary communities. The less original an individual is, the more easily he finds companions like himself. The philistine is welcome everywhere, because his needs are elementary and universally shared.

If the environment consists only of what acts upon a being, then the genius truly inhabits a broader environment than the philistine. The latter is shaped chiefly by what is narrow, local, visible, immediate, and present.

The genius, in addition, is influenced by what is cosmical, psychical, impersonal, remote, invisible, past, and possible. The philistine requires living authorities and concrete examples to change his behavior. For the genius, a mere hint or suggestion—

from nature, from books, from obscure or eminent individuals – is often sufficient.

Individuality and environment, ability and opportunity, are mutually dependent. Neither can be understood as a mere cause or a mere effect of the other. Individual differences and originality arise partly from environmental change; conversely, changes in the physical and social environment are brought about by individual peculiarities and by genius. Just as environmental influence must accumulate through heredity to stimulate original human thought and action, so the influence of genius upon society must also be cumulative. Innovation requires repetition: the efforts of successive geniuses and talents must build upon one another before transformation becomes real and enduring.

Independent Individuals and Social Vision

Psychically independent or relatively isolated individuals – those who, for one reason or another, are less bound by tradition, custom, external forms, conventions, and restless material pursuits – possess a wider and clearer view of both nature and human society. Without breaking entirely, like criminals, the insane, eccentrics, or purely instinctive beings, from the compact mass of humanity that advances slowly and blindly, they maintain a certain distance from it. From this position they gain perspective.

Such individuals perceive the possibilities offered by the physical environment; they remain open to its suggestions and lessons.

At the same time, they receive the impact of the blind strivings, aspirations, and latent tendencies of the social group – forces which, because of internal contradictions and the sheer weight of numbers, cannot pass beyond vagueness and desire into decisive change. In independent individuals, however, these same tendencies freely transform into real movement in a new direction.

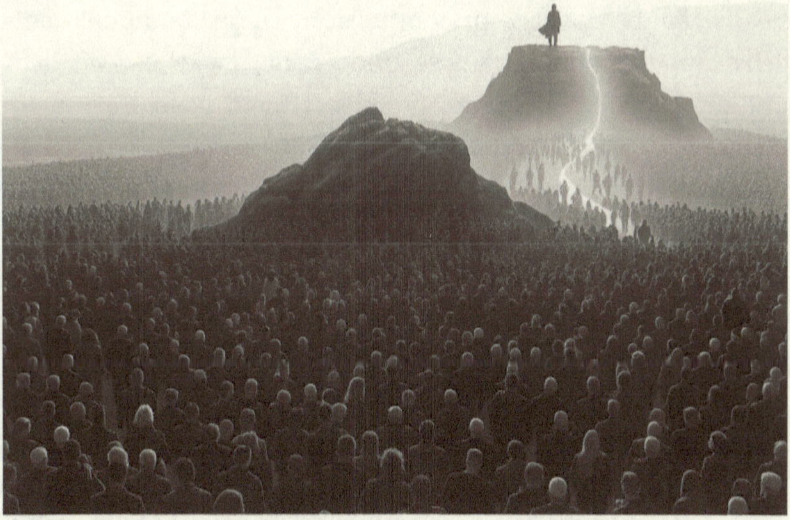

Semi-independent individuals, often closer in spirit to the independent than to the mass of philistines, soon follow, drawing behind them a greater or lesser number of dependent, imitative, mentally inert people. The larger body of humanity may persist in its habitual course and gradually decline, while a smaller, newly formed group slowly breaks its ties with the old order and follows a different, more advantageous, or more progressive path. In time, even this new group may divide again—into a smaller, more progressive section and a larger, more conservative one—and the process repeats itself.

Necessity and Genius

Neither individual necessity nor social necessity gives birth to genius. Their function is selection, not creation. Necessity encourages and favors useful originality; it prepares channels for the activity of genius and prescribes its direction, but it does not produce it. If necessity were creative, different races and nations confronted with similar needs would generate the same quantity and quality of genius—which they do not. At most, necessity acts as a secondary factor.

Abilities, originality, and genius are not products of aims, needs, wants, poverty, or compulsion. These conditions merely seize upon existing abilities, guide them, make use of them—and often distort, degrade, or deflect them from their natural course. Higher abilities—intellectual, artistic, moral—arise spontaneously whenever the lower abilities that serve bodily needs leave behind a surplus of mental energy. Geniuses commonly appear in families that either do not need to expend much energy on securing food, shelter, and social rank, or that choose not to do so. Inventors and creators are rarely greedy or acutely sensitive to material deprivation, and they seldom reap material rewards proportionate to their labor.

In modern society, where most people are forced to exhaust their time and strength in satisfying lower needs, higher abilities and genius remain the privilege of a small—and often degenerate—minority. In a truly socialistic society, however, where genuine solidarity and cooperation secure economic safety, leisure, and freedom for all, higher pursuits and genius will cease to be exceptional and dearly paid-for anomalies. They will become normal, widely shared attributes of humanity.

Our needs drive us to seize whatever best satisfies them and to invent new means for doing so. But only a surplus of energy—leisure, freedom from material anxiety and oppression—enriches life by enabling us to seek new aims, to cultivate new needs, or to develop those that exist only in embryonic form. A need never gives rise to new needs; on the contrary, each need strives to dominate the others and to harness all our abilities and energies to itself. Necessity is not the mother of great and genuine inventions; it is rather the exploiter of those inventions that promise usefulness and obedience. Greed and vanity encourage technical innovations that strengthen economic power, while moral and social ideas must struggle bitterly to survive. Genius invents not under pressure, but by freeing itself from pressure—by simplifying bodily needs and abandoning petty ambitions, thereby gaining the surplus energy required for creative work.

Historical Progress of Genius

It is well known that the average length of human life has increased not because vital energy has grown stronger, but because less of it is wasted—thanks to improved cleanliness, hygiene, and social conditions. The same is true of modern genius when compared with that of antiquity. The modern genius is not richer in native mental power; rather, he uses his powers more economically. He benefits from the accumulated knowledge of the past, from laws and formulas discovered by earlier thinkers, which allow him to survey vast fields of phenomena with relatively little effort, conserving his energy for further creation.

The superiority of the modern genius over the ancient, and of the educated genius over the uneducated, lies in this condensed transmission of human knowledge through schools, social groups, and family education. In the same way, humanity's conceptual thinking—its superiority over other intelligent animals—rests not only on greater innate capacity but also on social heredity, above all language, which enables learning from the experience of ancestors and contemporaries. Animals, by contrast, transmit experience almost exclusively through instinct and physiological inheritance. Even if it remains uncertain whether genius is increasing in sheer intensity or absolute power, there is no doubt that its range of interests, its field of action, and the number of those endowed with it are steadily expanding. Under a more just social order, humanity may one day consist largely of diverse forms of genius, mutually enriching, beautifying, and ennobling one another's lives.

Genius as Compensation

The presence of rudimentary organs, the muscular inferiority of civilized humans compared with their uncivilized ancestors, and of geniuses compared with philistines, as well as humanity's organic deficiencies relative to other animals, all point to one conclusion: intellectual progress is compensatory. It develops at the expense of the body. Inferior instruments of adaptation wither through disuse as superior ones emerge.

The uneven development of non-substitutable abilities speaks clearly for the compensatory origin of genius. The division of labor in social life makes it neither necessary nor possible for individuals to develop all their abilities equally. Without such division, society might produce talented people, but never geniuses. This explains the rarity of genius in rural life and its greater frequency in cities—though often accompanied by a decline in morality and solidarity.

Up to a certain point, there is no conflict between receptive and reactive mental abilities, no opposition between the intensity of special talents and the total range of abilities, no contradiction between the objective and subjective aspects of mental life. A balanced, continuous, many-sided development of mental powers may occur chiefly at the expense of the body—thinking at the expense of acting, intellectual refinement at the expense of physical strength or reproductive power. By contrast, an abnormal, one-sided, discontinuous development sacrifices one part of the mind to another: intellect at the expense of perception and feeling, or moral sentiment at the expense of clear thought.

In such cases, the strengthening of certain abilities proceeds hand in hand with the weakening, divergence, and disharmony of others.

Physiologically considered, it is not entirely incorrect to say that both genius and insanity arise from an overflow—a spilling over—of mental energy, whether caused by shock, obstruction, blockage of a channel, or by leakage. In the case of genius, this excess energy finds outlets in the higher centers of the brain and is transformed into creative, constructive activity. In insanity, by contrast, the same overflow, failing to discover such channels, produces devastation in both sensory and motor domains.

Unlike hierarchical social systems—which, if not transformed in time, inevitably see their ruling classes lose whatever usefulness they once possessed and degenerate into dangerous parasites, themselves succumbing to fatty decay while dragging the ruled masses into atrophic ruin—the individual organism represents the only hierarchical society in which the ruling class, namely the brain, is invariably concerned with the welfare of the whole. Even in the genius, the growth of higher brain functions, though occurring partly at the expense of the body, does not normally lead to degeneration or decay, except under extremely unfavorable conditions. Nor does it originate in degeneration, as Lombroso claimed. Rather, it replaces inferior physiological and anatomical modes of adaptation, as well as destructive and predatory capacities, with superior instruments—constructive and cooperative abilities, means of preventing waste of energy, and ways of compensating in quality and intensity for any reduction in mere quantity or extent.

Social and Economic Roots of Philistinism

The prevalence of philistinism in human society is not a natural necessity but the product of long-standing social and economic pressures. During the primitive nomadic and hunting periods, human groups lived in compact tribes or hordes characterized by uniform occupations. This external uniformity fostered internal, mental uniformity as well. At later stages, tyranny imposed by nomadic invaders, parasitic conquerors, and ruling castes upon both their own military forces and the subjugated agricultural populations tolerated no independent or critical judgment among the ruled.

In modern industrial society, economic dependence exerts a crushing pressure that extinguishes individuality by reducing the masses to mere instruments for increasing the wealth and comfort of a small group of idlers. These and similar forces—ultimately reducible to fear, whether direct or indirect intimidation exercised by crowds, leaders, or exploiters—paralyze mental spontaneity, at least in its outward expression. Only one motive force is left intact: instinctive or voluntary imitation.

As a result, humanity consists largely of philistines—automatic, thoughtless, empty-minded and empty-hearted individuals, intellectually blind and purely imitative—and of a considerable minority of semi-superior and pseudo-superior men who dare assert originality only in directions that serve, or at least do not threaten, the interests of their immediate social superiors: rulers, exploiters, monarchs, financiers, employers, capitalists, governments, churches, and organized parasitic professions.

If natural and physiological causes alone were at work, philistinism would be a rare exception. Fortunately, a number of subtle and often imperceptible factors are steadily weakening its grip: the increasing division of labor; the absence of rational solidarity among exploiters and even their mutual rivalries and denunciations; the growth of individual liberty through easier travel and urban concentration; the anonymity afforded by city life and the press; the willingness of modern industrial workers to sacrifice their own independence for that of their children and of the intellectual proletarians who enlighten the masses openly or indirectly; and the short-sightedness of exploiters who, in pursuing immediate gains, undermine the long-term interests of their own class and descendants. All these forces help to liberate humanity from paralyzing fear and from human parasitism—the deepest source of philistinism and social misery.

Social pressure weighs most heavily upon adults, and especially upon those who are normal and sane. Children and eccentrics are granted a somewhat wider margin of spontaneity. This may partly explain why hereditary philistinism becomes more evident after adolescence and why there are fewer philistines among children than among mature individuals. It also helps explain why genius appears more frequently in families marked by nervousness or eccentricity than in those characterized by placid temperaments.

The intellectual emptiness and degeneration often observed among the wealthy are not primarily acquired through power, privilege, idleness, or indulgence in pleasure. Rather, they are inherited from self-seeking, materialistic ancestors whose unrestrained greed destroyed or atrophied all higher human aims. Such ancestors at least possessed one driving purpose—the accumulation of wealth—which stimulated activity and indirectly connected them with certain forms of progress that could be exploited. Their descendants, whose fortunes increase almost automatically, often enter life without any aim at all, without natural interests upon which to expend their energy in a meaningful way.

Fear, Survival, and the Protection of Mediocrity

In nature, it is not always the strongest, bravest, or most progressive organisms that survive. Often the timid, weak, and unenterprising endure because they remain hidden, avoiding danger. Similarly, ignorance, stupidity, and frivolity protect many individuals from being crushed by exploiters, who reserve their hostility for competitors, critics, and serious-minded moral innovators capable of disrupting profitable systems of exploitation.

Only those proletarian geniuses who remain within the oppressed strata of society, confining their faint, self-generated light to the narrow boundaries of their own milieu, often escape corruption or persecution—much like deep-sea organisms that carry their own weak illumination in crushing darkness.

The Economic Basis of Misoneism

Aversion to change, new ideas, and reform—so often cited as an insurmountable psychological obstacle to progress—would amount to little more than a weak and harmless resistance if it were not reinforced by economic interests and by fear of financial loss or diminished prestige. Psychological inertia alone counts for little among normal individuals living under tolerable conditions; most people hunger, however vaguely, for change, new aims, and new sources of activity and enjoyment.

The same pseudo-rulers and captains of industry who violently oppose reforms advocated by socialists, moral innovators, and altruists become eager champions of those same reforms once resistance becomes futile and compliance can be simulated cheaply, without loss of power or wealth. Likewise, academicians and pseudo-scholars who scorn ideas originating outside professional or institutional circles readily embrace novelty once they can claim it as their own—or once they have silently appropriated it from some obscure and unprotected genius.

Economic interest, not mere ignorance or vanity, lies at the heart of most intolerance. Industrial magnates who remain unmoved by the destruction of countless lives in their enterprises proudly support causes such as international peace when these align with their commercial interests. Religious conservatism appears hostile to science only because religion is mistaken for its institutional shell. The Church, in reality, often functions as a parasitic body nourished by ignorance, superstition, and fear.

Thinkers such as Karl Marx and Achille Loria have convincingly shown that financial interests underlie intolerance toward pioneers of science, free thought, democracy, and new creeds, just as they motivate the obsession with titles, ranks, empty honors, ceremonies, and pomp. Philistine intolerance, by itself, is largely passive and psychological, rooted in suggestion and mental inertia. It turns into active persecution only when deliberately inflamed by pseudo-leaders whose economic interests are threatened by unpaid, genuine leaders of humanity.

The true reason rulers persecute independent, critical, and ideal individuals is not conservatism but fear. They tolerate inferiors who accentuate their own superiority, and they accept clever individuals who are submissive and mercenary. What they cannot endure are defenseless superior minds whose light exposes their emptiness, and whose independence unmasks the purely ornamental and self-assumed nature of their authority.

In sum, philistinism is not a natural destiny of humankind. It is a social product, sustained by fear, economic dependence, and parasitic structures. As these foundations weaken, the innate human capacity for independence, creativity, and higher development inevitably reasserts itself.

Conditions and Incentives

Pain— Pain is a stronger stimulus to thinking and creation than pleasure. From a social standpoint, it may act as one of the causes of genius; from an individual standpoint, it is primarily a stimulus. Over time, a social cause may be reduced to a personal incentive, just as an individual incentive may gradually assume the force of a cause.

Awakening from the inertia of thoughtlessness under the pressure of necessity is painful. In its earliest phase, thinking—when it serves merely to flee from unfavorable conditions—is accompanied by suffering. In its second phase, when it seeks better conditions, it becomes a source of pleasure. In the final phase, when satisfactory or favorable solutions are reached, thinking ends in indifference—just as the pre-thinking stage, the state of mental inertia, also began in indifference.

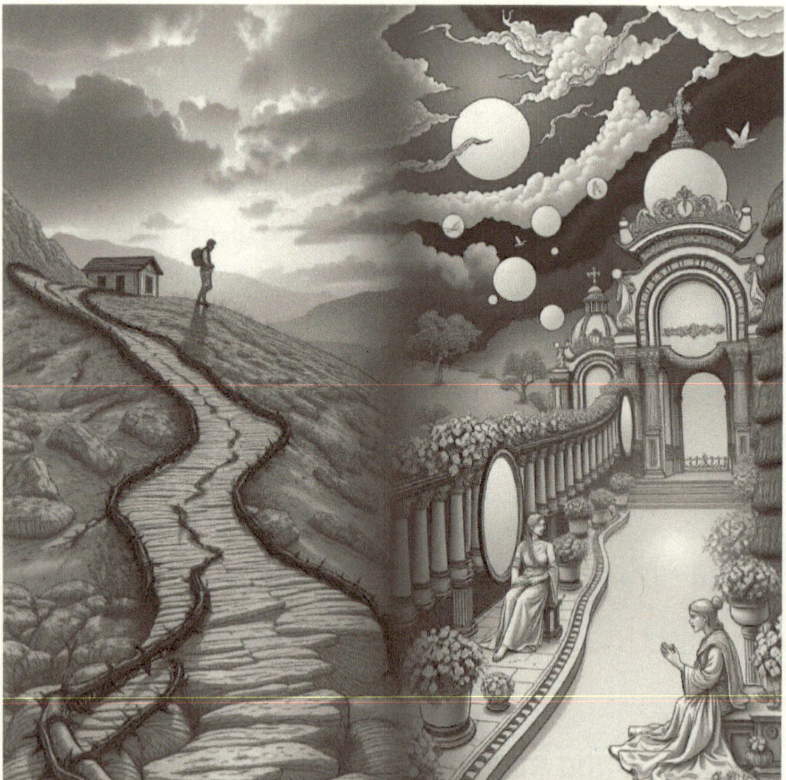

Poverty— It is often asserted that poverty stimulates thinking and creativity. This is true only within definite limits.

Just as temperature stimulates psycho-physical activity only within a certain range—paralyzing it below or above that range—so poverty may intensify originality only so long as it does not pass the point of insecurity and uncertainty regarding the satisfaction of the most elementary bodily needs. There is as little progress in equatorial regions as near the poles; likewise, there are as few geniuses among paupers as among the highest financial aristocracy.

Only the poor and socially obscure have real opportunities to perceive the predatory foundations of human society and the hideous inner lives of the so-called upper classes, because no one finds it worthwhile to wear a poetic mask in their presence.

Harsh reality forces itself upon those who must struggle against its asperities and thorny paths. Even one's true self becomes visible only when its wishes are resisted, its assertions disputed, and its impulses contradicted. The unprotected individual—thrown upon his own resources, relieved by no one of responsibility, compelled to foresee and calculate every step, and opposed in every effort at self-assertion—cannot afford to lose himself in reverie, dreams, delusions, mystical intoxications, or sweet thoughtlessness, as the rich so often do.

The path of the wealthy, smoothed by the self-multiplying power of capital and constantly ministered to by others, requires no sustained effort. Deprived of voluntary muscular or mental exertion, they easily fall prey to hypnotizing, morbid, and shallow literature, to flattering spiritual delusions, idle speculation, daydreaming, Christian Science, theosophy, and other forms of mysticism. Only the philosopher supported by the state, the church, or capital can afford to retreat into a narrow circle of shadowy ideas and deny or forget the existence of a harsh and stormy reality beyond. Only such a thinker can afford to blur the distinction between dream and reality, subjective and objective. In the struggle with nature, humanity gains clearer insight not only into the material world but also into the depths of its own soul. If to live means to struggle, to act, to overcome obstacles, to gain mastery over nature and oneself through knowledge, then the financial aristocracy—despite its glittering, noisy, and seemingly brilliant parade—does not truly live but merely vegetates. It becomes a crushing burden upon the laboring masses, who are worn out by unnecessary overexertion and compulsory drudgery designed solely to make the path of a negligible minority not merely smooth but dangerously slippery.

Both extremes—the desperately poor, who lack the strength and opportunity to struggle, and the excessively rich, who have nothing to struggle against—are doomed to mental and bodily degeneration. Both become obstacles to human progress. Geniuses and leaders of humanity arise mainly from the middle strata of society, where a relative economic independence exists, and where life is neither entirely free from struggle nor completely crushed by it.

To pursue higher intellectual aims seriously, one must have reached a certain bodily and economic stability. Lower needs must be satisfied regularly and rhythmically so that energy is conserved. One must be protected from economic fluctuations that demand constant, restless attention. In highly industrialized and commercial societies, such as the United States, people struggle so intensely against economic uncertainty that they no longer seek moral or intellectual elevation in theaters or lectures. They seek only amusement, relaxation, forgetfulness, thoughtless pleasure, and emotional intoxication.

Poverty and Intellectual Fertility

Necessity—not poverty—is the mother of invention. The struggle against poverty excludes the pursuit of truth. When poor geniuses are productive despite deprivation, this does not disprove the paralyzing influence of poverty; it merely shows that geniuses refuse to struggle against it in order to preserve their freedom for intellectual pursuits. Only when poverty becomes intolerable does the genius awaken from his habitual indifference and resist—if only briefly—before surrendering again. Instead of defending himself, he addresses threatening poverty as Archimedes addressed the Roman soldier: Noli turbare circulos meos (Do not disturb my circles).

Isolation and Social Life

The impulse to mental activity usually comes from without—from the cosmical or social environment—but the activity itself is strictly individual. To unfold fully, it requires prolonged isolation, interrupted only by occasional contact with nature and society, unless the initial impulse is strong enough to carry the process to completion unaided.

Excessive and continuous social contact prevents the formation of broad and accurate views of human nature and social relations, and renders resistance to unreflective suggestion impossible. Excessive isolation, on the other hand, blurs perception, drains vitality from thought, and gradually alienates the individual from everything human. Only a wise alternation and balance between isolation and association produces harmonious individuality. Entirely solitary beings and entirely gregarious ones alike remain unprogressive.

Such productive isolation becomes possible only in economically advanced societies and large cities, where the division of labor is highly developed and individuals are freed from the immediate pressure of the mass. In rural or primitive tribal life, rigid customs and inviolable traditions suppress originality everywhere except in despotic chiefs, unruly children, and the insane.

Division of labor depends in part on population density. The denser the city, the greater the chance for psychic isolation—

the chance to live less observed, less constrained, and less influenced by incongruent minds. At the same time, the chance of encountering congenial spirits increases. This combination strengthens the individual's courage to remain true to himself, to express his originality, and to give free rein to his natural inclinations.

Isolated individuals—human or animal—are thrown upon their own resources. Responsibility weighs heavily upon them, compelling self-control, inhibition, deliberation, complex thinking, foresight, learning from experience, and the selection of the most adaptive impulses. As members of a crowd, however, both humans and animals relapse into intellectual inertia, emotional exaggeration, automatic imitation, impulsiveness, and destructive mono-ideistic activity, devoid of introspection and foresight.

Between the critical, original thinking of the psychically isolated genius and the extreme suggestibility of the crowd lies the rationally imitative life of societies, parties, and associations, as well as the indirect self-suggestion exercised by public opinion through books and journals. The genius is constructive and progressive; the public is cooperative; organized societies are conservative; crowds are destructive.

The life of solitary or isolated animals is relatively simple. Their surroundings change little, and few unexpected events occur during their lifetime. Consequently, such animals require only a modest amount of brain work. By contrast, animals living in crowds or herds possess no real freedom of mind, no psychological space for individuality. Since foresight and responsibility rest chiefly with leaders, the mental activity of gregarious animals is reduced to a minimum—to imitation and docility.

Social life, however, offers a reasonable degree of psychological freedom while also imposing a tolerable share of responsibility upon each member. Contact among members of society is neither as close nor as compulsory, nor as rigid and personal, as that within a crowd or horde. Individuals endowed with strong, expansive, and original natures—who require greater freedom, solitude, and contemplation—must also bear a heavier burden of responsibility and discomfort. Leaders rarely tolerate, and still less protect, those who resemble or surpass them, especially critics who might eclipse their authority.

Although the responsibility borne by a gregarious social being is less than that of a solitary one, social life itself is far more complex and progressive. As a result, even protected social individuals are compelled to perform more mental work than isolated animals living purely by their own resources, if only through the imitation of influential figures. The greatest intellectual effort is demanded of independent individuals who keep their distance from the herd, as well as of genuine leaders—not sham or nominal ones who cloak self-preservation in the language of service. By leaders, we mean all superior individuals who guide or influence others, whether directly or indirectly, consciously or unconsciously.

From this line of thought arises the assumption that solitary animals of the same species tend to be nearly equal in intelligence, since each bears equal responsibility for its own survival and that of its offspring. Social life, on the other hand, distributes responsibility unequally, leading to a concentration of intelligence at the periphery—among the unprotected, the most responsible, and the most isolated.

This observation, however, does not justify the cruel competition of modern individualistic and capitalistic society, in which the majority exhaust their strength and intelligence in a hopeless struggle against insurmountable obstacles, while a minority—often intellectually inferior—enter life upon paths so smooth and effortless that they slide into degeneration, imbecility, or insanity. These privileged individuals decay because nothing restrains them from indulging excessively in those psycho-physiological functions that yield immediate pleasure.

The economic dependence inherent in capitalism binds together, compulsorily and indissolubly, individuals of widely differing abilities and aspirations. The more capable and idealistically inclined are thereby hindered in their upward course; they dare not advance or express opinions likely to provoke hostility, jealousy, or even indifference. In a socialistic society, where every individual enjoys the right to employment and is economically dependent only upon the community as a whole, intellectual progress would become easier, more widespread, and less hazardous. The more intellectual or altruistic individual would risk nothing by inviting others to follow the same path, since he could readily dissolve unproductive associations and seek out more congenial companions—or even withdraw psychologically, if his work were destined chiefly for posterity.

Close, intimate, and continuous association—between mother and child, between action and thought, between teacher and disciple—is both possible and necessary during early stages of development, marked by weakness, imitation, and simplicity of purpose. In maturity, however, such closeness becomes stifling and harmful. This later stage, characterized by strength, adaptability, initiative, and complexity, is better served by loose, voluntary, and intermittent association. It is not enough that individuals recognize their own interests; they must also possess the freedom to act in their defense. At present, the protection of general interests is best divided among thinkers, poets, and men of action. Those who act lack the leisure and originality to discern the deeper needs of humanity, while thinkers absorbed in discovering such needs often lack the patience for leadership and agitation. Only among primitive societies, pursuing simple aims, can one individual think, feel, and lead simultaneously. Such unity may reappear in a highly developed democratic society. Close and continuous association accelerates development among individuals who naturally move in the same direction. Between uncongenial individuals—those whose paths diverge—it becomes a source of tyranny, disturbance, and mutual obstruction.

Motion, variation, and spontaneity are the primary and original conditions of isolated beings, from unicellular organisms to atoms. Close and indissoluble aggregation, by contrast, breeds stagnation, inertia, imitation, and aimless oscillation. Yet as aggregates grow larger, regrouping and differentiation occur, restoring progressiveness on a higher plane. The once homogeneous group divides into smaller, loosely connected units, so that innovation no longer requires the approval of the entire mass but only of a sympathetic subgroup.

If bodily adaptability has reached its limits, it is partly because organs are too rigidly interrelated to change freely. Similarly, intellectual and psychological adaptability stagnates in small communities due to rigid social bonds, and in large cities due to economic dependence and oppression. Fear—of the majority in small communities and of a predatory minority in large ones—stifles originality. This fear explains why geniuses often avoid direct personal communication and instead address humanity from a distance, through books and the press.

The remedy does not lie in a return to primitive isolation or rural simplicity, but in the democratization of society—an ascent to a higher form of independence: voluntary isolation within society itself. True progress will be restored when mutual control and free exchange among social groups are established; when the people collectively serve as the ultimate judges of innovations affecting general welfare; and when a social order guarantees to every individual the right to work, a secure livelihood, and the freedom to change occupation or residence on the basis of personal ability and responsibility, rather than privilege, influence, or recommendation.

Division of Labor

The division of labor, which initially arises from inequality of talent or opportunity, soon becomes in turn a cause of increasing inequality and differentiation among human abilities and chances. By allowing individuals or classes of individuals to devote more time and energy to a single line of pursuit, it deepens both specialization and disparity.

In primitive communities, where all members shared the same occupations and were largely self-sufficient, a change occurred as soon as certain individuals—by virtue of greater talent or more favorable circumstances—began to produce certain things better than their fellow tribesmen. The less gifted or less fortunate then developed the desire to exchange a larger quantity of their own products for a smaller quantity of these superior goods. As population density increased and intercommunication between tribes grew, this demand strengthened. It encouraged the more gifted or fortunate individuals to abandon the production of goods they could easily obtain through exchange, and to concentrate instead on their preferred forms of production.

Unfortunately, with the rise of the division of labor and the exchange of values among producers, space was also created for a quasi-parasitical class of middlemen. Later still, when exchange was facilitated by the invention of money as a conventional medium and unit of measure, an even more dangerous predatory class emerged from within this non-productive group—the class of financial speculators. It is likely that the first individuals freed from the unprogressive condition of being jacks-of-all-trades were those who used their leisure to produce artistic works or articles of luxury. Next came those capable of producing useful objects of superior quality, or at least of giving them an artistic finish. Only in more recent times has the division of labor been degraded from a promoter of talent and quality into a mere instrument for increasing quantity—an instrument that renders industrial exploiters independent of, and dominant over, workers, and that stultifies, philistinizes, enslaves, and automatizes the masses.

Human and Animal Intelligence

The four-footed ancestor of man, by virtue of greater intelligence, gradually specialized his forelimbs for grasping and his hind limbs for locomotion and for bearing the weight of the body. Unlike modern apes, which occasionally rise on their hind legs only for specific purposes, this ancestor increasingly persisted in the erect posture, even when there was nothing to grasp or reach for. This persistence, though initially painful, likely conferred the advantage of a wider visual horizon and the ability to detect enemies at a distance.

To claim, as some anthropologists have done, that the erect posture caused human intelligence, or that the use of tools and machines made man intelligent, is misleading. We see men today who constantly use machines and become more stupid through mechanical repetition, while improvements in machines often come from those who use them less steadily, and entirely new inventions come not from machine-workers but from thinkers. Intelligence alone, of course, could not invent without material and suggestion from nature. Without observing animals clinging to floating trees, man would not have invented the boat; without caves or hollow trees offering shelter, he would not have invented the house. Yet while nature or chance suggests such rudimentary means, their refinement and transformation spring from intelligence alone.

This does not mean that intelligence created the erect posture. Rather, intelligence seized upon it and retained it after encountering it accidentally while the forelimbs were occupied, and because the hind limbs proved adaptable to supporting the body's weight. Mental energy cannot devote itself to distant and abstract aims before immediate and urgent needs have been met, just as a spring of water forms a river only after filling nearby cavities and overflowing them. To say that man used tools merely because his erect posture freed his hands is as inadequate as saying that a river exists only because the cavities it encountered were too small to contain it. Without sufficient potential energy, the water would simply form a lake.

To attribute human intelligence, civilization, and superiority over animals solely to the freeing of the hands is to deny any qualitative difference between human and animal mental energy. Such a view leaves both intelligence and the erect posture unexplained. Why did upright posture become a permanent trait in man alone? If progress depended merely on surplus energy, why do powerful animals waste their surplus in aimless play, while man directs it toward purposeful activity?

The more plausible explanation is that human intelligence possesses a higher potential—an inborn pressure, a restless dissatisfaction that seeks new goals. This elevated potential enables the human mind to rise from the purely sensational level typical of animals, to the perceptual level characteristic of the philistine, and finally to the conceptual level where superior intellects find their true home.

In the human species, racial experience is transmitted chiefly through education and social heredity rather than through rigid physiological inheritance. Human instincts are generalized, vague, and non-specialized, leaving room for individual adaptation, modification, and evolution. In animals, by contrast, instincts are well defined and highly specialized, leaving little scope for initiative. In them, not only habits but even single actions may become instinctive—organized into physiological mechanisms that are automatically activated whenever the original stimulus reappears. In man, the looseness of instinct is precisely what makes freedom, originality, and progress possible.

End of the Chapter

Chapter-3.
Types of Superior Minds and the Inner Hierarchy of Intelligence

This chapter maps the hidden architecture of superior minds, revealing how poets, scientists, technologists, and philosophers differ not merely in talent, but in direction, depth, and purpose. By uncovering an inner hierarchy of intelligence, it offers readers a lens for recognizing genuine greatness—and for understanding their own dominant ways of seeing, thinking, and creating.

Types of Superior Minds

Observation and Interpretation

Taken as a whole, the various types of genius differ from the class of average individuals chiefly in degree; yet among themselves, and in contrast with intermediate types, they differ in kind. What all geniuses share is a power of combination and creative imagination, though this power manifests itself in different proportions and directions.

Observation is most essential for scientific creation, while interpretation and explanation are the chief requirements of philosophical work. The technical and artistic genius possesses a maximum capacity for observation, together with a constructive imagination built upon it. The philosophical genius shows a maximum power of interpretation. In the scientific genius these two abilities—observation and interpretation—are more evenly balanced. The distinctive faculty of the technological genius lies in the clear perception and imaginative grasp of movement, that is, of correlated relations of space and time. From a large number of observations, the scientist draws a few conclusions; the merely talented scientist draws conclusions that are less general than those of the scientific genius. From a small number of observations, the philosopher draws many conclusions, or conclusions of a higher degree of generality than those of the scientist.

The genuine, inborn observer observes spontaneously and involuntarily, without conscious intention, without preconceived hypotheses, and without reference to the satisfaction of intellectual or bodily needs. His observation is disinterested. The subsequent elaboration, digestion, and interpretation of the material thus gathered, however, is voluntary and purposeful, imposed either by himself or by others. The opposite holds true of the genuine speculative thinker. Beyond the minimum of observation required as a basis, his further observations are guided by interest, intention, and will, serving chiefly to confirm or refute theories that arise in him spontaneously.

Because the philosopher's mental vision is adapted to wide horizons and bird's-eye views rather than to details, he is liable to a kind of intellectual farsightedness. The scientist, accustomed to attending to particular phenomena and narrow generalizations, is correspondingly prone to intellectual shortsightedness and to a contempt for broad syntheses—often born of an inability to attain them. Excessive metaphysical speculation leads to a form of mental presbyopia; excessive positivism leads to mental myopia. Each extreme is the counterpart of the other.

The philosopher is only indirectly interested in particular facts; he values them insofar as they allow him to ascend to general views. His primary concern is the relation and harmony between things rather than the things themselves. For the scientist, and still more for the technologist, generalizations are chiefly means to a clearer understanding or more effective use of particular facts.

The objective, positive, experimental thinker approaches men and things from without. He displays a maximum activity of perception and a minimum of reasoning, that is, a minimum activity of the associative and combinative centers of the brain. He tends to reify human beings, blurring the distinction between vital and mechanical phenomena. He advances from the simple to the complex by adding and synthesizing elementary properties. He refrains from forming hypotheses when sense data are insufficient, and he is uneasy at rising above facts on a weak empirical foundation. His preferred dwelling place is the sober region of concrete facts and actualities, and his originality lies mainly in the discovery of new facts.

The subjective or speculative thinker, by contrast, approaches everything from within. He shows a minimum of observation and a maximum of interpretation and combination. He tends to humanize things and animals by attributing to them an excess of human qualities. He proceeds from the complex—his own inner life—toward the simple through abstraction, subtraction, and analysis. To him, disconnected and unexplained facts are intolerable; his mind requires theories to hold them together. His natural habitat is the elevated, poetic realm of abstract concepts and general views, and his originality lies in devising new theories that embrace facts discovered by observers or dimly anticipated by himself.

Each of these two types tends naturally to ignore or dislike the other, unless compelled by public opinion or professional necessity to take notice. Both, however, admire the rare genius who unites observation and speculation, and who knows how to learn from both observers and theorists alike.

Subjective or humanistic speculation is especially liable to corruption when pressed into the service of egoism, commercialism, or profit-seeking. A notable example is pragmatism, which merely renames the old sophistic doctrine that man is the measure of all things. It is therefore unsurprising that this philosophy gained prominence in societies dominated by commercial standards. One may hope that thinkers of less predatory traditions will resist the spread of such morally distorted doctrines.

Impressibility

The poet is more impressible but less clear in consciousness than the thinker. He portrays the world and the soul as they impress him under particular psycho-physical conditions. The scientist, by contrast, describes the world as it impresses him under relatively constant and normal conditions.

In ordinary circumstances, the philistine is scarcely impressed by anything outside the sphere of bodily needs. The artist and the technologist, on the other hand, are impressed by certain aspects of reality at the expense of others. The artist, in the narrow sense—poet, painter, sculptor—responds primarily to emotional and aesthetic qualities; the technologist to practical and utilitarian ones. The scientist and the philosopher attend more to harmony itself: the scientist to partial harmony and relative truth, the philosopher to total harmony and absolute truth.

Sentimentalism and Thought

Youth, unaware of life's obstacles and human meanness, looks forward with sentimental hope; old age, weakened in body and mind, looks back with sentimental admiration upon an idealized past. The prosaic individual, finding little poetry in real life, becomes sentimental when life is represented on the stage or in fiction. In all these cases, sentimentalism signifies one-sidedness. Thought, by contrast, is many-sidedness; the prosaic attitude is affective blindness.

Sentimentalism consists in the mind dwelling long upon a few things or aspects of things. Thought moves more freely, dwelling briefly on many aspects. Opposed aspects awaken opposed feelings, which partially neutralize one another and free the mind from narrow sentimentality.

Just as there is no force without matter, nor matter in absolute rest, so there are no sentiments without ideas, nor ideas without a sentimental aspect. Sentiments are the motion of ideas; ideas are psychical matter in motion. Excessive emotional shock produces confusion, dissociation, or disintegration of mental functions and hinders the formation of clear ideas. Moderate emotional stimulation, however, invigorates thought and facilitates the combination and fusion of ideas.

Emotion and idea are not separate mental states but inseparable components of a single state, combined in varying proportions. Emotion is the centrifugal, dynamic element; idea is the centripetal, stabilizing one. As ideas gain clarity and meaning through richer associations, emotional explosiveness diminishes. Conversely, when ideas are isolated and poorly connected, emotional intensity and impulsive discharge increase. The frequent association of strong emotion with vague ideas has led some psychologists to suppose that emotions are merely obscure ideas, overlooking the fact that many confused ideas exist without any significant emotional accompaniment.

Vague and inarticulate longings, drifting aimlessly across the stormy inner sea of the sentimental soul—simple, undifferentiated states of mind in which emotion predominates and the ideational element is almost extinguished—find their most fitting and most beautiful expression in music, including dance or acted music. Music is therefore the lowest and most primitive of the arts, and for that reason it is the favorite art of women, children, and philistines.

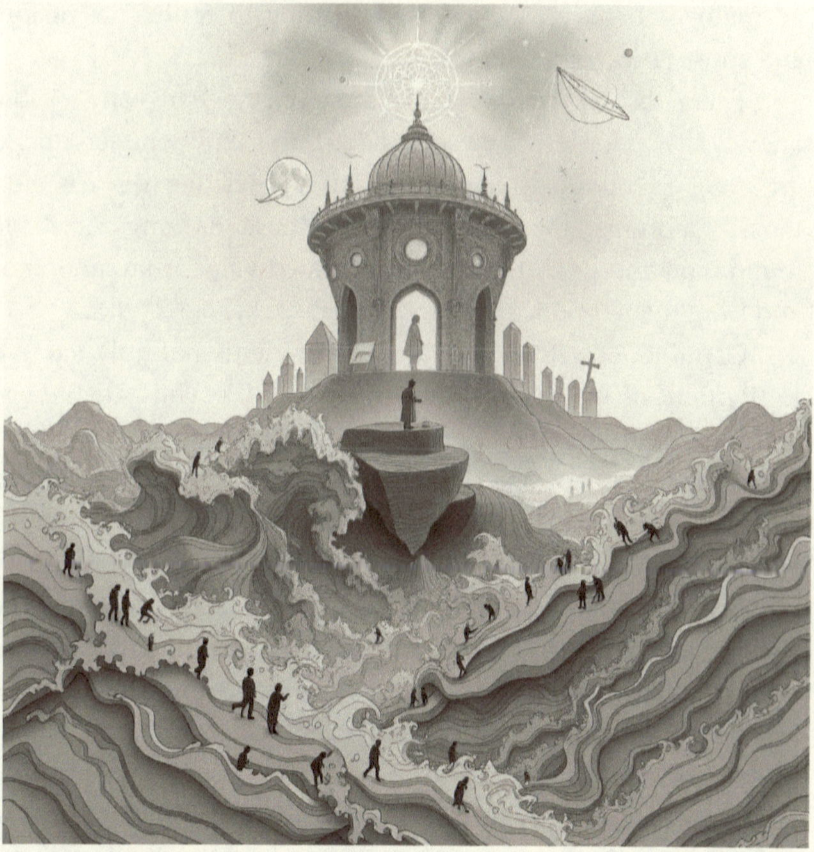

As states of mind grow more complex, as the cognitive element gains clarity and differentiation, and as the impetuosity of emotion diminishes, higher forms of art come into play—sculpture, painting, poetry, drama, and the novel. When the cognitive element becomes dominant and emotional intensity is reduced to a minimum, the most adequate forms of expression are science and philosophy.

Mysticism—including spiritualism, occultism, theosophy, and related tendencies—occupies an intermediate position between pure emotionalism and clear thinking. It may represent either an ascending stage toward lucid, original thought, or a descending stage of decay into confused emotionalism. In mystical modes of thought, the boundary lines between related or analogous concepts are erased, leading to confusion, fusion, and substitution of meanings.

There is no fundamental antagonism between reason, knowledge, science on the one hand, and emotion, sentiment, art, religion on the other. Increased knowledge dispels only those emotions that are illusory—those lacking objective foundation and deriving their exaggerated value from ignorance and from the hypnotic suggestions of those who exploit it.

Genuine, objective, and useful sentiments not only survive in the light of truth; they flourish more fully. Thus, the atheist who rejects divine sanctions of morality and future rewards or punishments is not less moral or altruistic than the religious believer—often he is more so. The naturalist, physician, or scientist who studies the human body in all its naked reality is no less capable of love than the ignorant person. The psychologist who can no longer idealize parents or children does not love them less, but loves them more sanely and steadily. The love of the enlightened mind is sober, enduring, and free.

Science does not attack or destroy genuine or metaphysical religion—that is, the cosmic sense of belonging to the universe as a whole; the feelings of awe and wonder before infinity; the humility inspired by the fragility and transience of human life. Science attacks only superstition, fear, ecclesiastical absurdities, and religious exploitation. Reason does not annihilate instincts; it renders them adaptable, modifiable, and serviceable. Knowledge and truth are not hostile to sentiment; they are hostile only to error, illusion, fetishism, and ungrounded belief.

Mature, reflective thought does not coexist with youthful, explosive enthusiasm. There is no cause for regret in this, for such enthusiasm is unstable and unreliable—it either remains inactive or overshoots its aim.

No amount of theological sophistry can conceal the irreconcilable conflict between science and anthropomorphic religion, especially as expressed in prayer and ritual that invoke supernatural intervention. Science advances human progress by teaching mastery over nature through knowledge; prayer is a relic of primitive magic, a symbolic discharge of desire coupled with a vain hope of influencing natural events.

In short, just as parasitic social institutions, fraudulent reputations, and absurd customs can survive only by avoiding public criticism, free discussion, and comparison with useful institutions—seeking instead secrecy, darkness, taboo, and repression—so too do harmful emotions, phobias, parasitic ideas, hypnotically implanted beliefs, and bad habits thrive only by avoiding consciousness, self-examination, and reason. They seek refuge in the darkness of the subconscious, in isolation, and in ornate or opaque language.

Subject-Matter and Method

The subject-matter of art, in its widest sense (including useful arts), consists of the harmonies and conflicts between desire and reality or knowledge; its aim is beauty or utility. The subject-matter of science is knowledge itself; that of philosophy is the harmony of different kinds of knowledge or the underlying reality they express. Science and philosophy aim directly at truth and indirectly at utility.

A practical art is a system of useful, perceptual, concrete, particular, and implicit knowledge. An esthetic art concerns emotions, passions, and states of mind together with their outward expressions. A science is a system of explicit, verified, conceptual, general knowledge. Philosophy is the highest and most comprehensive system of conceptual knowledge, dealing with both mind and cosmos. The artistic sense represents the earliest and lowest stage of unselfish human interest: a vague, emotional, undifferentiated concern with nature and humanity. The scientific and philosophical spirit, by contrast, embodies clearly defined, intellectual, and unselfish interest in the essence of the universe.

When we perceive an object for the first time, we cannot distinguish what belongs to the object itself from what belongs to its surrounding context. Only through repeated experiences—seeing the object in varying situations and emotional settings—do we learn to separate the objective from the subjective, the essential from the accidental. We then become capable of recalling the object independently, using it for classification, thought, and reasoning rather than mere reverie.

Unique, unclassified, emotionally charged experiences belong to memory and imagination. Recurrent, typical, and communicable experiences belong to knowledge and thought. The artist deals with the individual, exceptional, subjective, and emotionally colored elements of experience. The thinker deals with the general, objective, recurrent, and communicable elements—experience stripped of its accidental and incommunicable features.

In art, knowing and doing are inseparable and mutually reinforcing. In literature, science, and philosophy, knowing is differentiated from doing; it sets aims but does not prescribe every action. Literature presents relations implicitly through particular cases, while science emphasizes variable relations between phenomena. Philosophy seeks beneath surface diversity the enduring, unifying essence of things—beneath historical and political noise, the slow currents of psychological and economic truth. Much of the professorial and academic talk about method is little more than empty rhetoric. Thinking and investigating cannot follow single, isolated methods. Analysis presupposes synthesis; induction presupposes deduction; experimentation presupposes hypothesis. All conscious activity is guided by ideas. Only in exposition can methods be artificially separated; in genuine thinking and invention, such simplification is impossible. The primary method of art is synthesis. Analysis plays only a secondary role and is employed chiefly in the service of broader and richer syntheses. In science, the reverse holds true: description and the concrete lead the way toward explanation, generalization, and abstraction. In philosophy, both methods are equally indispensable. Synthesis in art and philosophy is constructive: it creates concrete or abstract organic wholes. Synthesis in science, by contrast, is primarily classificatory: it orders phenomena so that they may be more easily handled, and thus prepares the raw material for higher forms of synthesis. Analysis places in our hands the inert matter—the substance, the body, the anarchic elements of things and of ideas—but it allows their collective movement, their associative energy, their inner spirit of cooperation, to escape. Art recombines the scattered elements of cosmic and human reality into new wholes that are more beautiful or more useful. Philosophy, in turn, unites the disconnected concepts of science into a more or less coherent, consistent system capable of illuminating and guiding life. What the psychologist, the scientist, or the philosopher expresses explicitly in abstract form, the artist and the technician express implicitly in concrete form—whether in a living work of art or in a mechanism of far-reaching usefulness.

Point of View and Aim

Art views the world from a single point of view; science approaches it from an indefinite number of viewpoints; philosophy strives to embrace it from infinitely many perspectives, sub specie aeternitatis. Art achieves subjective truth, in the form of beauty or utility. Science attains objective but relative truth. Philosophy seeks objective and absolute truth.

Primitive art represented the world successively from many points of view, and therefore lacked perspective and coherence. Modern art views the different parts of a whole simultaneously from a single standpoint. The artistic mind does not confuse unconscious inferential corrections of perception with immediate sense data; it distinguishes clearly between what is given by the senses and what is added by imagination and intellect. In its psychic combinations, it does not lose sight of the constituent elements.

What applies to the artist in the realm of perception applies, mutatis mutandis, to the scientist and the philosopher in the realm of concrete or abstract concepts.

First Cause and Ultimate Result

The first cause and final aim of art, science, and philosophy is normally a general intensification of psycho-physiological rhythms—and, in abnormal cases, a compensatory and one-sided intensification. Art produces this intensification directly: through a single sense in the lower arts (music, dance, color), or through several senses combined with lower intellectual functions in the higher arts. This effect is powerful but transient. It arises and subsides almost immediately with the stimulus, often throwing the individual into ecstasy, exaltation, or self-forgetfulness, and rendering him temporarily docile to the influence exerted upon him.

Rhythmic intensification produced by coarse dance, intoxicating music, or other physical and emotional stimulants—religious, sexual, gambling, or self-deceptive practices—is unstable, uncontrollable, and unfit for constructive purposes. It represents an easy but inadequate reaction against mental stagnation and frustrated development, and it is commonly followed by a swing toward exhaustion, inertia, and weariness of life. The rhythmic intensification associated with science and philosophy is modest but enduring. It is communicated indirectly, appears slowly, and may never entirely fade. It enriches the individual, awakens aspiration, and makes him a willing collaborator with his teachers and kindred minds. Science brings the individual into harmony with the world as it is; philosophy aligns him with the world as it tends to become.

Philosophy—understood as genuine, self-created thought rather than mere scholastic repetition—tunes the human mind to infinity and eternity. It raises the individual above the turbulence, narrowness, and discouragement of everyday life; above fragile hopes and ungrounded fears.

Physiologically, a normal intensification of vital rhythms is marked by an increased demand for better nourishment and for a richer field of activity. Psychologically, it is indicated by optimism, by a state of well-being, or at least by sustained hopefulness. Science, as a rule, directs its attention chiefly to divergence, dissimilarity, and differentiation among phenomena—dissecting, separating, and distinguishing. Philosophy, while not denying these distinctions, seeks their underlying unity and meaning.

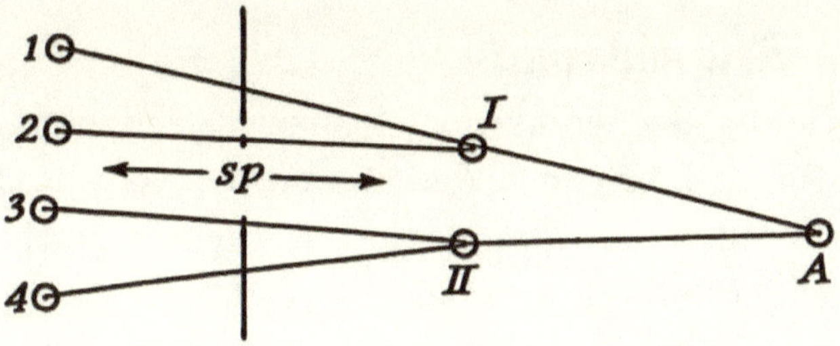

The fundamental method of art is synthesis. Analysis plays only a subordinate role and is employed chiefly for the sake of broader and more comprehensive syntheses. In science, the relation is reversed: description and attention to the concrete prepare the way for explanation, generalization, and abstraction. In philosophy, both analysis and synthesis are equally essential. Synthesis in art and philosophy is constructive: it creates organic wholes, whether concrete or abstract. Synthesis in science is primarily classificatory: it arranges and orders phenomena so that they may be more easily handled, and thereby prepares the material for higher unifying efforts.

Analysis places in our hands the inert matter of things and ideas—their substance, their elements, their bodily structure—but it allows their collective movement, their associative energy, and their inner spirit to escape. Art recombines the scattered elements of cosmic and human reality into new wholes that are more beautiful or more useful. Philosophy, in turn, unites the isolated and disconnected concepts of science into a more or less coherent and consistent system capable of illuminating and guiding life. What the psychologist, the scientist, and the philosopher express explicitly and abstractly, the artist and the technician express implicitly, through a concrete body—either in a living work of art or in a mechanism endowed with wide-reaching usefulness.

Point of View and Aim

Art views the world from a single standpoint; science approaches it from an indefinite number of standpoints; philosophy strives to comprehend it from infinitely many perspectives, sub specie aeternitatis. Art attains subjective truth, expressed as beauty or utility. Science attains objective but relative truth. Philosophy seeks objective and absolute truth.

Primitive art represented the world successively from many points of view, and therefore lacked perspective and coherence. Modern art views the different parts of a whole simultaneously from one consistent standpoint. The artistic mind does not confuse unconscious inferential corrections of perception with immediate sensory data; it clearly distinguishes what is given by the senses from what is added by imagination and intellect. In its inner combinations, it does not lose sight of the elements out of which they arise.

What holds true for the artist in the sphere of perception applies, with appropriate modification, to the scientist and the philosopher in the realm of concrete and abstract concepts.

First Cause and Ultimate Result

The first cause and final aim of art, science, and philosophy is normally a general intensification of psycho-physiological rhythms—and, in abnormal cases, a compensatory and one-sided intensification. Art produces this intensification directly: through a single sense in the lower arts such as music, dance, and color, or through several senses combined with lower intellectual functions in the higher arts. This effect is powerful but transient. It arises and subsides almost immediately with the stimulus, often throwing the individual into a state of exaltation or self-forgetfulness, and rendering him temporarily receptive to external influence.

The rhythmic intensification produced by coarse dance, intoxicating music, or other physical and emotional stimulants—religious, sexual, gambling, or self-deceptive practices—is unstable and uncontrollable. It is unfit for constructive purposes, represents an easy but inadequate reaction against mental stagnation, and is commonly followed by exhaustion, inertia, and weariness of life.

The rhythmic intensification associated with science and philosophy is modest but enduring. It is communicated indirectly, appears slowly, and may never entirely disappear. It enriches the individual, awakens aspiration, and makes him a willing collaborator with teachers and kindred minds. Science brings the individual into harmony with the world as it is; philosophy aligns him with the world as it tends to become.

Philosophy—understood as genuine, self-created thought rather than verbal or scholastic repetition—tunes the human mind to infinity and eternity. It raises the individual above the turbulence, narrowness, and discouragement of everyday life; above fragile hopes and ungrounded fears.

Physiologically, a normal intensification of vital rhythms is indicated by an increased demand for better nourishment and for a richer field of activity. Psychologically, it manifests itself as optimism, as a state of inner well-being, or at least as sustained hopefulness. Science, as a rule, directs its attention chiefly to divergence, dissimilarity, and differentiation among phenomena—dissecting, separating, and distinguishing. Philosophy, without denying these distinctions, seeks their deeper unity and enduring meaning.

There is no conflict, no real antagonism, between specialization and comprehensive knowledge, or philosophy. The truly profound specialist ultimately becomes a philosopher, or at least develops a philosophical outlook; and the genuinely objective philosopher often ends by concentrating his attention more deeply upon one particular field than upon others. The former arrives at philosophy through the gradual acquisition of breadth; the latter attains objectivity by confirming, through concrete knowledge, what was at first only an intuitive sense of proportion—the sense of the unequal and relative importance of the various domains of human endeavor.

The specialist begins by focusing his interest upon a single science. As he advances further and further into the domain of his chosen field, he inevitably comes into contact with neighboring sciences, and gradually with more distant ones. At a later stage, he begins to suspect, and then consciously to seek, an underlying harmony among all fields of knowledge. What starts as concentration thus ends in integration.

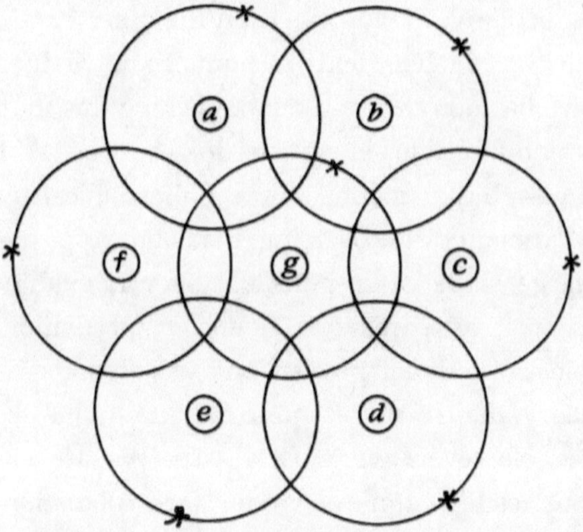

The polyhistorian or the philosopher follows the reverse path. He begins with many points of view, with a wide diffusion and dissemination of interests. He gathers knowledge simultaneously from various domains. As his partial familiarity with each field increases, patterns emerge, relations become visible, and a philosophical system gradually takes shape.

Every science—and psychology in particular—is a pathway that leads toward the heights of philosophical contemplation. The contempt for philosophy sometimes expressed by certain scientists does not arise from superiority, but from limitation. It is the attitude of those who have not advanced far enough along the difficult, laborious, and demanding road of their own specialty to glimpse the broader horizon beyond it. Their disdain for philosophy springs from the same source as the fox's contempt for the grapes he could not reach: an unconscious confession of frustration rather than a judgment of value.

There is a real antagonism between superficial specialism and dialectical, speculative philosophizing. The superficial specialist does not know his own field deeply enough to perceive the countless lines of connection between his specialty and the domains of other specialists.

The speculative philosopher, on the other hand, knows too little about the concrete fields of human knowledge to discover an objective harmony among them. Lacking this foundation, his indolent mind fabricates imaginary links between scattered ideas and mistakes these fictions for a philosophical system. This dialectical, romantic, ideologizing, parasitical type of speculation bears a large share of responsibility for mental poverty and confusion—just as parasitical financial speculation is largely responsible for economic poverty and social bondage.

In theory, there is no reason to halt at ultimate explanations; in practice, however, we must do so. We are compelled to restrain our restless, aimless craving for explanation—a relic of primitive imagination and a relapse into the wandering habits of animistic thought—just as the wanderlust of tramps echoes the roaming instincts of our nomadic ancestors.

The purely speculative philosopher resembles a scientific tramp and parasite. Just as the regulations, discipline, and complex machinery of economic life weigh intolerably upon the tramp, so the norms, methods, preparatory training, and patient labor of science weigh upon the speculative philosopher. He prefers to roam freely in the realm of imagination at the expense of experimental workers, much as social parasites live at the expense of manual laborers.

Nomadic wanderlust could once be indulged with impunity while vast regions lay uninhabited or weakly defended; and parasitism will become impossible in a truly just society where working classes govern their own affairs.

In the same way, pure metaphysics will become impossible when every science undertakes the task of working out its own metaphysical implications—after establishing a firm experimental foundation.

To do justice to genuine, ideal metaphysicians, however, they should be compared not to tramps but to explorers of unknown and polar regions. They too possess wanderlust, yet they subordinate it to higher aims: the exploration of the obscure and uncertain realms of metaphysics. The poorly equipped speculator either perishes in these regions or returns bearing nothing but the phantoms of his own fear-exalted imagination. The verbal or pseudo-metaphysician, meanwhile, never reaches those uncharted territories at all, yet returns with greater noise and self-advertisement than the true explorer. The antipathy felt by scientific specialists toward philosophers thus has its parallel in the resentment of settled, routine people toward adventurous nomads.

Intellectual Hierarchy: Classification

The Man of Action

From an intellectual standpoint, the pure or ordinary man of action does not stand much higher than the philistine. As a rule, he is a pseudo-intellectual and often a pseudo-moral figure. Although mercenary historians and credulous masses erect monuments to him and celebrate his memory, the impartial student of human nature cannot assign him a high rank in the hierarchy of mental abilities. Human progress would be more continuous and far less disturbed if thinkers—genuine superior minds—exercised direct intellectual guidance over society. The man of action depends upon the ideas elaborated by thinkers; the thinkers, if given the choice, could dispense with the former's mediation, though not with that of technologists, but only with leaders, statesmen, professional reformers, and organizers.

The pure man of action is defined by ceaseless activity. Restlessness is his life. Solitude, contemplation, reverie, or thinking for its own sake terrify him—especially thought that cannot be immediately translated into action. His mental activity moves in simple, unbranched circuits leading straight to muscular discharge. His knowledge of people and things is empirical and practical, never theoretical or general. He does not care for the "why," only for the "what." He wants to know how to act quickly and effectively, how to provoke reaction, how to manipulate outcomes—not to understand underlying physical or psychological laws.

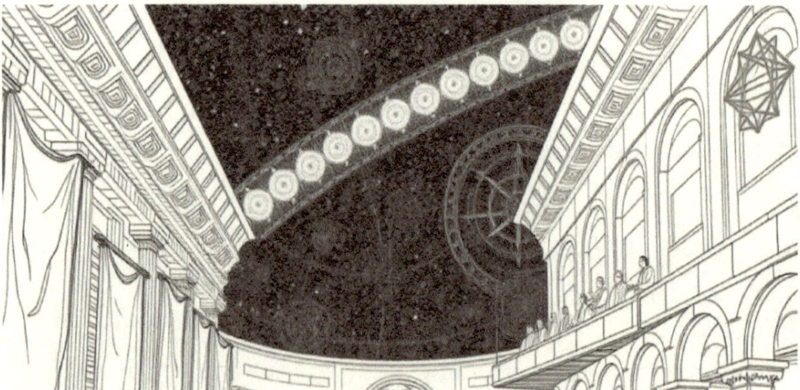

If he is a leader of men, his concern is limited to what pleases or displeases them, what excites them, what secures their confidence, and how they can be used. Whether he exploits them for material gain and vanity, or mobilizes them for causes that flatter his altruistic self-image, his ability to lead does not prove genuine understanding. On the contrary, a true understanding of human nature would temper his enthusiasm. If he grasped the insignificance of personal immortality and the smallness of human struggles within the vast, eternal processes of the universe, he would be less impulsive and more restrained.

The technologist or physically active worker understands the material he acts upon better than the social leader understands the people he commands. For both, knowledge is merely a means to an end. Excessive, deep, or general knowledge would hinder them; hence they avoid it. They tolerate science, art, and philosophy only insofar as these serve their immediate aims. When social thinkers cooperate with social organizers, it is not from ignorance of the latter's hostility to intellect, but from the recognition that such cooperation may help create conditions of greater leisure and freedom—conditions under which intellectual life can flourish.

The man of action is necessarily one-sided, limited in ideas, even mono-ideistic. One cannot pursue many practical aims as one can entertain many lines of thought. To realize and preserve a single practical objective requires constant vigilance and uninterrupted exertion—especially in a society distorted by ruthless competition. Practical pursuits forbid interruption, demand fixation on details, and require direct engagement with people and things. The larger and more ignorant the mass acted upon, the greater the danger that it will fall under the control of unscrupulous leaders whose so-called executive ability consists of flattery, intimidation, intrigue, and bribery.

The contrast between active and contemplative men is often not a division between types but between degrees. The so-called active type consists of those who feel compelled always to be doing something—anything—rather than thinking or waiting; who prefer immediate action, even at the risk of later undoing it, over careful planning; who seek visibility and attention; who learn only by doing and only what can be directly practiced. The contemplative type, by contrast, is not inactive, but deliberate. He acts rarely and only after weighing means, consequences, and lasting value. He lacks patience for routine execution and does not content himself with merely practical knowledge.

The man of action acts frequently and achieves little; the thinking man acts rarely, but his actions are enduring and far-reaching. Left to themselves, the thinkers and philosophers of humanity would long ago have achieved the peace, culture, and universal brotherhood that men of action have promised—and failed to realize—throughout history.

Poet and Thinker

From an evolutionary point of view, the thinker or philosopher must be regarded as superior to the pure poet. Sentimentalism is characteristic of immaturity; it represents a transitional phase in intellectual development, whereas scientific and philosophical thinking belong to maturity. If we accept that the development of the superior individual recapitulates and anticipates, in condensed form, the evolution of humanity as a whole, we are led to the conclusion that art in general, and poetry in particular, correspond to a lower stage of development than science and philosophy.

The thinker may, at times, descend again into the warm and fertile regions of poetry; and the poet or artist may occasionally rise into the clearer and calmer realm of philosophical reflection. Yet despite flashes of profound intuition or insight, the poet remains, as a rule, an immature, confused, obscure, inconsistent thinker. Even the most philosophical of poets does not constitute an exception to this rule.

The poet represents a primitive form of thinking. He thinks in images rather than in concepts, and therefore expresses his thoughts in pictorial language. He grasps the general and the abstract through the particular and the concrete; he interprets the new, the inanimate, and the impersonal in terms of the old, the traditional, the animate, and the personal. Because conflicting images, unlike conflicting concepts, cannot coexist in consciousness but only succeed one another, the poet's mind tends to be partial, one-sided, unstable, and sentimental.

Juvenile and Mature Types

Psychical maturity is marked by a rapid and comprehensive grasp of wholes and multiplicities, and by the capacity to conceive the abstract, the essential content, and distant ends. Psychical juvenility, by contrast, is characterized by a clearer and more objective perception of parts, details, concreteness, form, and immediate aims.

What holds true for maturity and juvenility in ordinary individuals applies equally to the different types of superior men. In comparison with the scientist and the philosopher, the artist represents a more juvenile type. Within each category, the same distinction reappears.

An artist who emphasizes detail and form belongs to the juvenile type of his class; another who stresses conception and unity becomes a philosopher-artist and belongs to a maturer type. An exclusive emphasis either on form or on idea is a symptom of extreme immaturity or of decline. Theology, in this sense, represents either the juvenile or the senile stage of metaphysics.

The tenth step in a series does not require more energy than the preceding ones; it merely demands greater effort because the general level of vital energy has declined.

Yet the tenth step cannot be taken before the ninth. The same principle applies to mental processes. Abstract thinking does not consume more energy than concrete thinking, but the concrete must precede the abstract. To begin with the concrete and advance toward abstraction presupposes a richer, more developed, and more mature intellect than remaining forever confined to concreteness.

The immature novelist or dramatist seldom goes beyond the fairy tales and fantastic stories of childhood. At best, he repeats—often with slight modifications—what he has heard from gossip or read in books. He depicts people and events from the outside, concentrates exclusively on one or two individuals as though the rest of humanity scarcely existed, and either ignores reality altogether or reproduces it indiscriminately, like a photographic film, burdened with trivial and accidental details. If he possesses some introspective ability, he portrays a single emotion or pursuit as though it absorbed his hero's entire existence.

The mature psychological or philosophical novelist and dramatist, by contrast, penetrates beneath appearances. He scrutinizes his own inner life and understands the souls of many types of men. Behind individual characters he reveals broader human types and social classes. While describing particular lives, he opens vistas of general life-conceptions; while dealing with present or past events, he hints at future developments. He illuminates the complex structure of society even when focusing on a single stratum. His sense of proportion enables him to distinguish the vital from the trivial, the instructive from the irrelevant, causal connections from mere coincidence.

Classification and Intellectual Interests

A hierarchical classification of superior minds cannot be based solely on the predominance of particular mental functions, for all mental functions are involved in every genuine act of thought. Nor can it rest simply on the balance between observation and speculation. Speculation is not the distinctive mark separating philosopher from scientist, for both rely equally on hypothesis and assumption. The experimental chemist employs as much implicit speculation in his analyses as the social reformer does in his ideal reconstructions. The physiological psychologist who ridicules philosophical psychology often fails to recognize that he too constructs unverifiable theories in his measurements and analyses.

Both science and philosophy begin with observation, proceed through hypothesis, and return to observation and experiment to test and revise those hypotheses. The real difference lies not in the presence or absence of speculation, but in the complexity of the problems addressed. The philosopher, endowed with a broad intellectual horizon, refined interests, bold aspirations, and a wide mental grasp, attacks problems of great complexity. The scientist, with narrower aims and fewer intellectual needs, confines himself to simpler, more immediate, and more manageable domains.

Mental superiority also cannot be classified solely according to dominant abilities such as observation, memory, imagination, or reasoning, without regard to underlying aims and interests. We observe and remember most readily what aligns with our dominant concerns. Thus, one individual may notice in an instant what another would overlook for hours—not because of superior faculties, but because of different interests. The philosophically minded person, concerned with enduring values and broad perspectives, is often indifferent to transient facts, gossip, conventions, and trivialities.

What distinguishes scientific from non-scientific observation is not speed or accuracy alone, but the guiding interests and the nature of the subject matter. The same holds true for introspection. The psychologist is not necessarily more introspective than others; rather, he attends selectively to those inner states that possess general significance. The poet remembers emotions; the psychologist remembers the thoughts they provoke. The psychiatrist is alert to deviations from the normal; the ethical psychologist is sensitive to the intrusion of selfish motives. In every case, inborn and persistent interests serve as the central point of reference, shaping perception, memory, and thought. In this way, the ascent from poetry to philosophy mirrors the ascent from immediacy to reflection, from image to concept, from youth to maturity, and from partial vision to comprehensive understanding.

When certain individuals are called observers, this does not imply that their mental activity is limited to mere seeing or recording. They also recollect, imagine, conceive, reason, and theorize. The distinction lies elsewhere: in the observer, all these mental operations are subordinated to observation and placed in its service. The thinker, by contrast, observes—or makes use of the observations and experiments of others—in order to reason upon them, to employ them as stepping-stones toward higher standpoints, broader perspectives, and more general conceptions. What distinguishes the observation of the thinker from that of the pure observer is that, for the latter, observation is an end in itself; for the former, it is a means—an instrument for testing earlier hypotheses and for stimulating the formation of new ones. To the pseudo- or professionally superior man, knowledge, art, and morality are merely tools for advancing personal interests. To the genuinely superior or vocationally devoted individual, they are ends in themselves, and only secondarily—if at all—means of gaining money or fame.

Food, shelter, clothing, and material possessions are ultimate aims for the philistine; for the intellectual individual they are merely means. To the technologist, mathematics, physics, and chemistry are methods for achieving and verifying practical results. To the mathematician, physicist, or chemist, technical constructions are embodiments of scientific principles, useful illustrations of theory rather than final goals. To the linguist, a nation's literature may serve chiefly as a means of discovering linguistic laws; to the cultural historian, language itself becomes a means of accessing literature and the intellectual heritage of peoples.

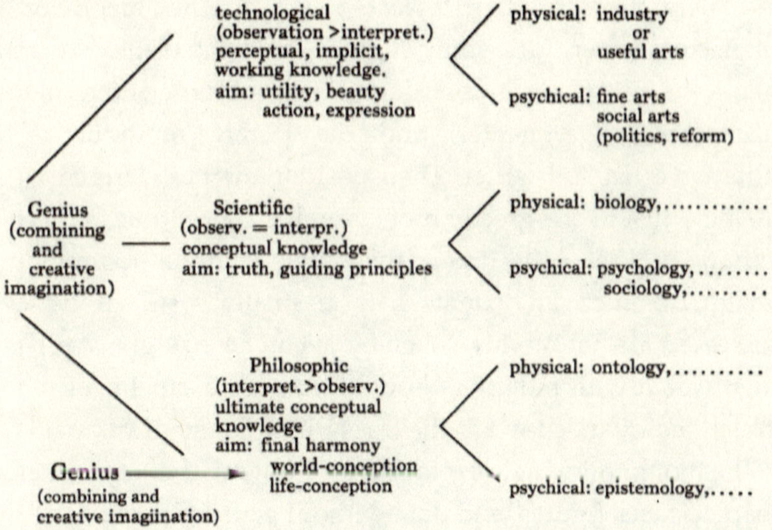

Whoever is deeply interested in a subject or in certain problems inevitably develops an interest in the methods by which those problems are approached, formulated, solved, and applied. Thus a scientist who lacks a natural inclination for mathematics or logic may nevertheless acquire a clear understanding of these disciplines once he feels the need to apply them within his own field. Conversely, the mathematician or logician, for whom mathematics or logic are not methods but ends in themselves, may fail to apply them effectively to complex domains that do not engage his interest. Yet even such a specialist must retain some concern with simpler or more general problems as a means of illustrating and grasping his own methods.

For science, art and technology function primarily as means—ways of discovering, expressing, and utilizing knowledge. Science itself, in turn, becomes for philosophy a means rather than an end: a stepping-stone toward ultimate truth, toward the presumed unity or underlying reality that lies beneath the diverse and fragmented domains of scientific knowledge.

Hierarchy.—At the lowest level of the hierarchy of intellectual superiority—only slightly above the plane of average men—we must place the thoughtless observer, the merely mechanical experimenter, and the purely reproductive or imitative artist and writer. Their position may be clarified by an analogy. Just as the greedy money-maker concentrates his entire activity and capacity upon the single aim of accumulating wealth, to such an extent that he finally loses—if he ever possessed it—the ability to enjoy what he has amassed, and must watch with bitterness how others, more capable of living, stretch their hands toward the treasure he has so dearly paid for; so the thoughtless observer and the empty-minded experimenter heap up facts, figures, and data without pausing to digest even a portion of them. They imagine—or profess to believe—that the more enormous their accumulation of raw observations becomes, the more easily knowledge will one day be extracted from it.

Yet the opposite occurs. Their minds end by losing—if they ever possessed—the capacity to assimilate and transform the intellectual wealth they have gathered. Much to their dissatisfaction, they are compelled to hand over this undigested material to younger, more creative minds—thinkers who possess the power to draw nourishment, meaning, and genuine enjoyment from it.

The purely observational, extrospective, descriptive, and experimental intellectual type lacks a deep, comprehensive, and many-sided thirst for knowledge. Were such a thirst present, it would be impossible for him to confine his mental activity for long periods—often for an entire lifetime—to a single narrow class of objects. His attention is ordinarily directed, not by inner necessity or intellectual passion, but by academic or popular fashion. In this way, he becomes a collector rather than a knower, a custodian of facts rather than a creator of understanding.

Within the field of observation itself, a genuine difficulty arises when we attempt to determine who occupies the higher place in the intellectual hierarchy: the observer of pathological phenomena or the observer of normal conditions—for example, the psychiatrist versus the psychologist proper. On the one hand, the authentic observer, who does not remain satisfied with superficial descriptions and who does not rest content with vague, shadowy, speculative notions of the essence of things and processes, is naturally drawn toward the pathological field. In abnormal or exaggerated conditions, the essential and distinctive features of phenomena often stand out more clearly, as in a caricature. On the other hand, it requires a higher degree of genius to discern the essence of things in their normal, everyday condition, where it is concealed beneath familiarity and apparent simplicity. The main body of those commonly called geniuses is composed of scientists and technologists; the vanguard consists of philosophers; the rear is formed by poets and artists. Or, stated more accurately, talented men make up the bulk of this army, while true geniuses constitute its leaders and officers.

Poets, insofar as they are poets, preserve and revive the past; scientists and technologists embody the present in its unfolding movement; philosophers anticipate the future. They are the first to catch—however briefly—the glimpse of ideal beauty and absolute truth that is granted to mortals.

It scarcely needs emphasis that nature recognizes no rigid classifications and no fixed lines of demarcation. There are no absolutely pure thinkers, no absolutely pure poets, and no entirely isolated types. The difference between a thinker and a poet lies chiefly in this: what is rule and purpose for the former is exception and accident for the latter, and vice versa.

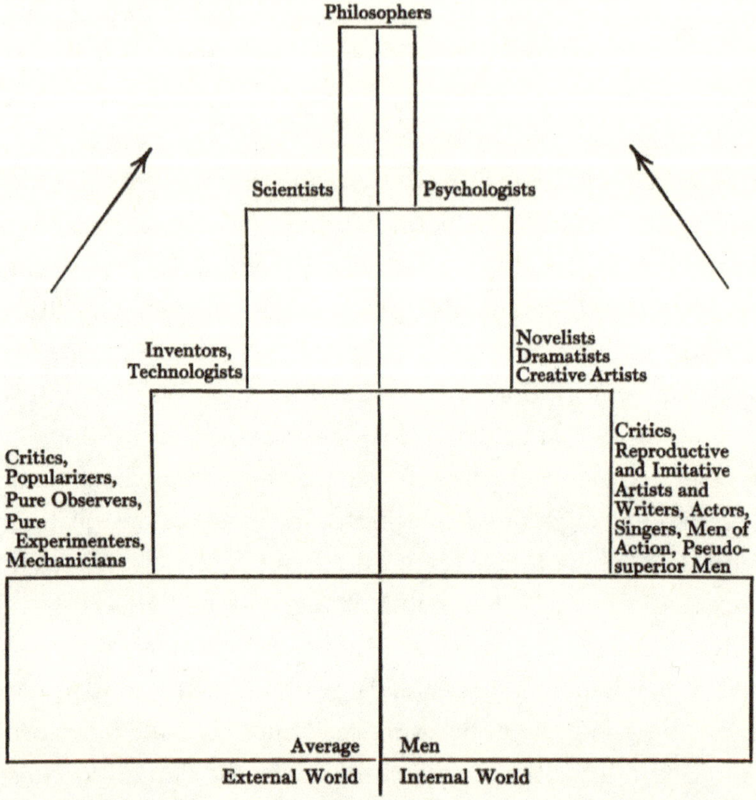

The poet, in comparison with the psychologist, stands in the same relation as the practical man does to the scientist. The psychologist observes his own mind directly and the minds of others indirectly, in an impersonal, objective, disinterested, and impartial manner; the scientist does the same with respect to the external world. The poet or artist, by contrast, observes his own soul and that of others for the sake of emotion, and therefore in a subjective, partial, and personal way. Similarly, the practical man notices the external world only insofar as it serves his immediate interests. To the psychologist, concrete situations are merely means—illustrations or raw material—from which abstract laws and general principles are extracted. To the poet, ideas are means for animating concrete situations, for giving life and character to a figure or hero: they form a hidden framework that supports a living creation, a scaffold upon which an idealized social world is built.

As we ascend from artists and technologists to the highest class—that of philosophers—the motor or action-oriented aspect steadily diminishes in favor of the sensory and contemplative aspect. Those rich in ideas tend to be sparing in action. This fact suggests the view that psychical energy may be physiological energy accumulated in a latent state; emotional energy would then represent a highly condensed and explosive form, while cogitational energy would be a more steadily available, organized form of cerebral potential.

Between two individuals who possess the same degree of many-sidedness, the more active especially the experimentalist—is superior to the less active, purely speculative type. Between two individuals of equal activity, superiority belongs to the one who is more many-sided. Yet, because division of labor is the prevailing rule, we rarely encounter an experimenter who does not borrow his initial ideas from a speculative thinker; and the latter, in turn, looks to the experimental work of others for confirmation of his intuitions.

The genuine speculative thinker (excluding the dialectical, parasitic, or intellectually dishonest type) is too rich in original ideas, too elevated and many-sided in his interests, to devote the necessary time and patience to experimentation and to the exhaustive pursuit of details and consequences. The experimenter, by contrast—especially the mechanical experimenter, who occupies in the intellectual realm a position analogous to that of the manual worker in the economic world—is often too poor in original ideas, too limited in inner intellectual impulses and needs, to relinquish easily any idea he possesses, whether it be a rare inspiration or one adopted simply because it is fashionable. For him, it is easier to probe ever more deeply into the same narrow field than to venture into a new order of problems. Hence the saying deserves to become proverbial: too much of an experimenter to be a deep thinker.

Curves of development

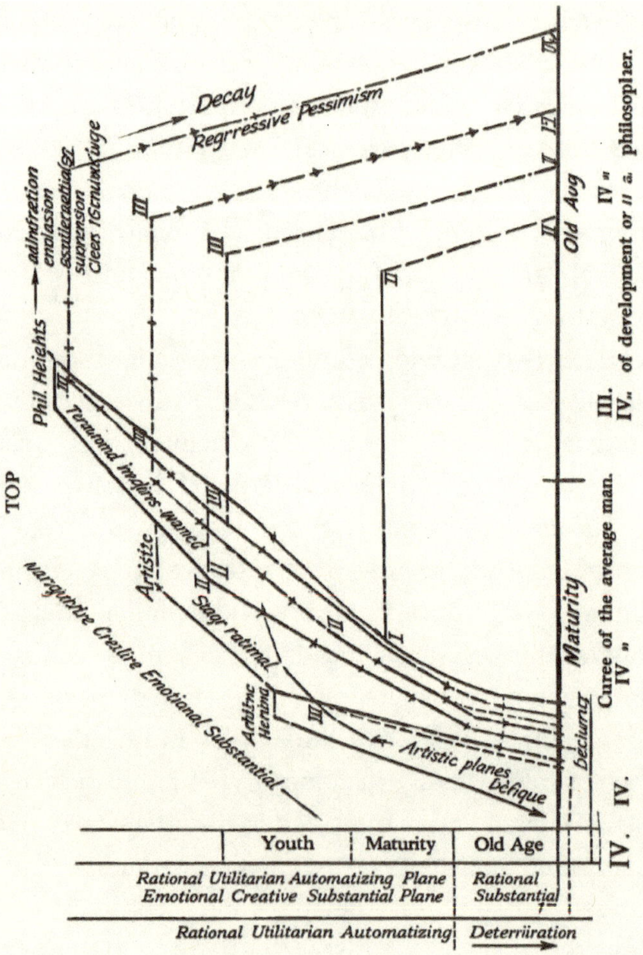

Without corroboration by the patient, conscientious scientist, we could never distinguish the fertile speculation of the genius from the idle constructions of a lazy mind, nor genuine intuitive insight from the mere guesswork and verbal fantasies of a superficial speculator. Conversely, without a guiding speculative idea, the scientist himself would never know what to observe, what to select from the chaos of facts, or upon what to experiment. Speculation and verification are thus mutually indispensable: each corrects, sustains, and completes the other.

To the moral genius, no single, fixed position can be assigned within the hierarchical scale of talent and intellect. He may appear at any level. He may be intellectually a philistine; in that case, his morality expresses itself chiefly in direct action, in concrete help rendered to particular individuals. He may be an artist, poet, or novelist; then his moral impulse manifests itself in the sympathetic portrayal of the oppressed and disinherited, awakening in us attention, compassion, and cooperative feeling. He may be a scientist—an economist, sociologist, or psychologist—or a philosopher; in that case, his morality takes the form of a relentless search for truth concerning social conditions, and of systematic efforts to devise ways of increasing social happiness and reducing human suffering. What unites all these forms of moral genius is not their intellectual rank, but their common aim: the growth of social solidarity and collective well-being. They differ only in method and medium—some act directly through personal influence and reforming action, others indirectly through art, literature, science, or philosophy.

Curves of Development.—The artist advances beyond the average individual chiefly along the lines of receptivity, observation, and reproduction. The scientist and the philosopher, by contrast, advance farther along the lines of creation and interpretation. In the genius, mental and bodily development do not run in strict parallelism, as they do in the normal philistine; the rhythms of growth are more complex, uneven, and differentiated.

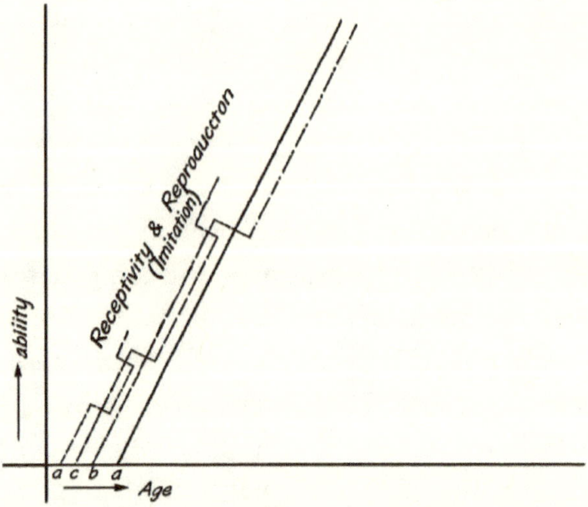

Scientist and Philosopher: Realistic and Romantic Thinkers.—Just as we perceive objects more clearly when we anticipate them, or when we have had similar perceptions before, so we understand general statements and conclusions drawn by others only when we ourselves possess incipient, vague tendencies toward the same generalizations, or have undergone comparable concrete experiences. Distant objects are practically non-existent for those who have not followed their movement or directed their attention toward them; likewise, highly general or philosophical statements remain empty sounds—mere mental shadows—for those who have not traversed the concrete experiential paths leading toward such abstractions, or who are unaware of the experimental and factual structure supporting them. All genuine scientific avenues ultimately lead toward the same summit of philosophical vision. Whichever scientific path one follows, the highest philosophical outlook reached is, in principle, identical. If philosophers often disagree, it is because many halt exhausted on the slope, or rest on a lower summit accessible from only one avenue, mistaking it for the highest point. Others, having climbed higher, lose sight of the lower levels altogether; the concrete experiences that once supported their ascent fade and become mentally non-existent. Such thinkers are often known—by a charitable euphemism—as idealists. The realist alone, even when standing on the highest subjective, introspective, and conceptual ground, retains a living connection with the lower objective, extrospective, and perceptual levels from which thought must ultimately draw its nourishment.

In this continuity—from observation to speculation, from fact to vision, from individual suffering to collective morality—lies the true order of genius: not a rigid hierarchy of isolated types, but a living, interdependent system in which science, philosophy, and moral purpose sustain and illuminate one another. The realistic philosopher—that is, the philosopher who rises to ever higher points of view and thereby embraces ever wider horizons, yet never loses sight of concrete realities, of particular individuals, actions, events, and struggles encountered in the lower regions of everyday life—alone is capable of assigning to everything its true place and significance within the total field of human and extra-human activity. Only such a thinker can judge proportionately, by constant comparison between the great whole and its smallest parts.

Only this philosopher can warn the philistine against the danger of allowing himself to be wholly and forgetfully absorbed in trivial, short-lived pursuits; in loud but empty, artificial, and perishable spectacles devised by exploiters; while remaining blind to approaching catastrophes that arise from unchecked human parasitism. Only he can recall the intellectual proletarians to the real, fundamental economic and ethical problems that must be solved before all others, and thereby save them from being entangled in fictitious, shallow, nebulous, formalistic, and truth-avoiding philosophies that serve capitalistic interests rather than human welfare. Among modern philosophers, the only one who, in my judgment, fully deserves the title of a genuine, consistent, steadfast, many-sided realistic philosopher is Max Nordau. That the caste of academic, state- or capital-supported philosophers largely ignores him is due to his plebeian manners, his love of independence, his non-official and non-technical style, his plain, unguarded, and unsparing language, his lack of grandiloquent scholastic verbosity, and his open disregard for time-honored, school-sanctioned doctrines and authorities. Wundt, despite his great abilities, remains too much a hair-splitter, too concerned with reputation, too eager for the applause of professional philosophizers, too deeply entangled in the nets of academic-capitalistic philosophy, and too absorbed in the display of erudition and the systematization of inherited doctrines, to rise to a genuinely realistic world-conception. Spencer, on the other hand, lacked the lived experiences of the proletariat needed to remain faithful to the philosophical and sociological realism of his earlier years.

Only the realistic philosopher is able to perceive the chaotic conditions prevailing both in the intellectual and in the economic world—conditions in which fundamental, life-sustaining activities are neglected, poorly rewarded, or even despised, while unessential, playful, childish, useless, and sometimes harmful pursuits are indulged, publicly financed, socially honored, and extravagantly rewarded. A thinker may be realistic in philosophy, individual psychology, or cosmological science, and yet remain unrealistic, romantic, ideologistic, and nebulous in sociological, political, economic, or ethical-psychological matters. The reason is simple. In the former domains there are no inherited privileges: every thinker must begin with personal observation and experience, with sensations, and gradually rise to perceptions and then to broader concepts. In the social, political, and economic domains, however, ready-made fictitious concepts and spurious ideals are imposed from childhood upon members of the privileged classes, depriving them of any genuine acquaintance with the predatory foundations of the social structure.

Only the intellectual proletarian is in a position to study human society as a whole, from its base upward, and to fully grasp its defective and unstable condition. He is born into the lower strata, which daily bear the crushing weight of uncertainty, hardship, and oppression; yet, by virtue of superior intellect, he can gain access—physically or mentally, through experience or reading—to the upper strata as well. Thus he is able to unravel the subtle causal connections between the simplified, brutalized, harassed existence of those at the bottom and the increasingly refined, complex, privileged, dream-laden, and effortless life of those at the top. If such a thinker is also a moral genius, he will never lose sight of humanity's vital needs and fundamental problems, even after attaining personal security. Unlike thinkers born into privilege, he will not allow himself to be carried away by sociological abstractions, political fictions, or grandiose but empty dreams. What has been said of the sociological realism of the intellectual proletarian applies, though in reversed sequence, to the impoverished middle-class thinker—Karl Marx, for example—and to the temporarily or permanently disinherited and persecuted aristocratic thinker—Peter Kropotkin, for instance. Beginning life among the privileged, they were later driven into the ranks of the struggling proletariat, where they learned to correct, deepen, and complete their world-conception, and to perceive men and institutions in their true proportions and significance.

End of the Chapter

Chapter-4.
The Inner Laws of Creative Life

This chapter reveals how superior minds differ not just in talent, but in kind. It explores poets, scientists, technologists, and philosophers as distinct intellectual types, and shows how depth of vision, integration of abilities, and range of understanding determine true intellectual rank and lasting influence.

Imitation and Creation

Imitation and creation do not stand in opposition to one another. The distinctive character of an individual, a nation, or a race reveals itself just as clearly in what is imitated as in what is created independently—just as much in the suggestions received as in those exerted upon others. Suggestion by itself can only intensify or weaken, hasten or delay, awaken or arrest, combine or separate mental processes that already exist potentially or actually within the individual who is influenced. It cannot supply what is wholly absent. It cannot give sight to the blind, thought to an empty mind, or feeling to an empty heart.

For this reason, it is as one-sided and immature to explain identical or similar myths, customs, beliefs, and practices found among distant races and tribes solely as products of contact, diffusion, and imitation, as it is to explain them solely as independent, spontaneous creations and as proofs of an absolute identity of human souls everywhere.

Not only truth and knowledge, but also error, illusion, and belief arise from the observation of real phenomena and real objects. The difference lies in the fact that error and illusion are built upon incomplete, inaccurate, second-hand, or emotionally clouded observations. There is no error, no belief, no legend, no myth that does not contain at least a small kernel of fact or truth, however deeply concealed. All creation, all original work, rests upon and contains a certain measure of imitation. All speculation must take its point of departure from observation. The human mind cannot create anything entirely from within itself without being aided, stimulated, and fertilized by suggestions coming from external nature.

Even music—the most purely subjective of the arts—draws its inspiration not only from the human heart, with its passions and longings, but also from the vast and powerful orchestra of nature itself: the wind howling in caverns and sighing through pine trees, the reeds whistling, waves moaning, rivulets laughing, thunder pealing, oceans roaring; the sounds of shifting sands and rushing waters in coral caves; the wild concerts of animals, the songs of birds and insects; the crashing waves against rocks; and finally, humanity's own spontaneous cries of emotion.

The genuinely original individual remains original even when he attempts to imitate and believes himself to be doing so. His originality asserts itself against his own will. Often at personal cost—since originality is mistaken for obstinacy or arrogance and therefore irritates those who lack it—he discovers that he differs from others, though he may not fully understand or appreciate this difference himself.

The pseudo-original individual, by contrast, imitates while believing he creates. In extreme cases, he cherishes originality for its own sake, without regard to the substance to which it is applied. The affected originality of the pseudo-superior individual is directed toward success rather than truth. Such a person is original in form, in trivial details, in words, while imagining himself original in substance and thought. Verbal or formal originality exhausts itself in inventing large words for small ideas, obscure or roundabout expressions for ordinary, simple, everyday facts. It attempts to conceal barren platitudes beneath ornate, picturesque language, much as one seeks to charm not by inner worth but by borrowed finery. Philosophical, broadly human, socially valuable truth, on the other hand, is too elevated to require decorative linguistic display.

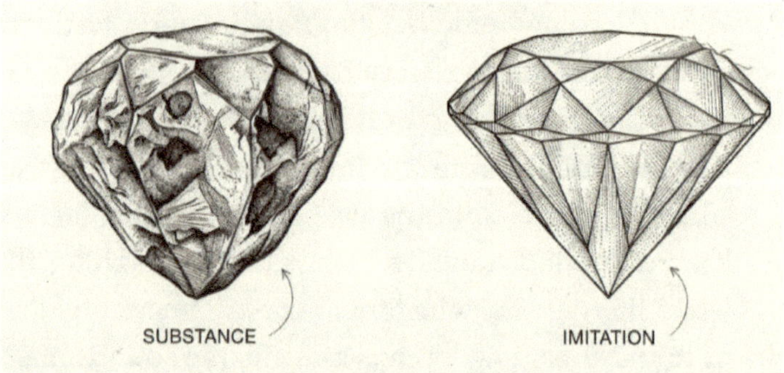

Verbal originality often repeats the same idea in many different forms, thereby creating the illusion of thoroughness; or it gives an old, commonplace truth a new outward form, which causes it to be mistaken for a new discovery. Genuine originality, in contrast, expresses many new and fertile ideas through one and the same linguistic form. Richness of thought, novelty of conception, and intellectual fertility frequently coexist with a simple, even monotonous style. Conversely, great stylistic variety and verbal abundance often accompany poverty of ideas and the monotonous repetition of the same commonplaces. As with people, so with ideas: ordinary, empty-minded individuals often parade in brilliant and fashionable attire, and commonplace ideas often circulate in imposing, scientific-sounding language.

Originality in some domains presupposes imitation in others. Originality in ideas, in essence, in the conception of ends rarely coincides with originality in form, detail, and means—and the reverse is equally true. No one can be a teacher in all things without first being a disciple in some. The speculative thinker is original in ideas, ideals, and aims; the experimental innovator may be original in methods, applications, and realizations. The former excels in broad views and large syntheses; the latter in discovering details and conducting analyses. The former grasps many aspects at once; the latter many details of a single aspect. One surveys from above, the other examines at close range. One seeks relations, causes, and meanings; the other facts, effects, and consequences. One perceives unity within multiplicity; the other multiplicity within unity.

From a vast mass of vagaries and nonsense, a small but precious quantity of fertile truth can sometimes be extracted. Yet this delicate task requires a mind trained in clarity, penetration, breadth, and critical judgment. To others, the rare and subtle truth—almost buried within endless layers of metaphysical confusion—slips away, leaving in their hands nothing but residue and obscurity.

The truly original individual approaches with reluctance the task of merely reproducing, popularizing, compiling, or commenting upon the work of others. When his strength lies chiefly in creation and explanation, he will not excel in imitation and description. As a rule, the knowledge acquired through reading and formal education serves the genius only as a catalyst. It stimulates and encourages his own thoughts to emerge, combine, and generate new creations, without itself being directly absorbed or consumed in those creations.

The premature craving for originality and intellectual wealth leads many into serious errors. It tempts them to mistake tautologies for explanations, verbal resemblances for real similarities, and artificial distinctions for genuine differences. Under this impulse, reality is often falsified half-consciously, patient verification is avoided, and theories without any solid foundation are hastily produced. Such pseudo-original minds forget that what appears as a small flash of originality is very often the final result of long, laborious observation and experience—just as a tiny quantity of gold is extracted only after immense masses of ore have been processed. An original idea that seems to spring suddenly from a single observation may, in truth, have been slowly prepared by many earlier observations stored in the subconscious. That single observation is merely the last, almost negligible weight that tips the balance and lifts a long-hidden idea into consciousness.

Both the premature yearning for originality and the decrepit yearning for it—that is, the craving no longer, or not yet, accompanied by the power to create—manifest themselves in many characteristic ways: indulgence in physical or emotional intoxicants; addiction to paradox for its own sake; a spirit of contradiction; philosophical negativism; obsessive hunting for verbal originality and unnecessary neologisms; ignoring, belittling, or ridiculing the genuine originality of others; persecuting contemporary truly superior men; excessive sensitivity to criticism and therefore anxious avoidance of it, except when it can be used for publicity; semi-conscious, self-deceptive plagiarism; and the counterfeiting of ideas through the coining of new words.

As an illustration of pseudo-originality in philosophy, one may point to the leading representative of modern sophistry, Henri Bergson. He identifies, merges, and confuses concepts which the human mind has learned, with great effort, to distinguish. For him, space and time become identical; spirit is reduced to pure duration; intelligence is equated with pure space; the physical world is described as merely inverted psychical reality. At the same time, he takes dishonest advantage of the fact that the same ideas can appear under different names. By combining such names, he gives the illusion of offering explanations and new truths, while in reality he merely presents tautologies and empty phrases. By suggesting that different names represent different ideas, he simulates a richness of thought that he does not actually possess. Among the terms with which he juggles—different in sound but identical in meaning—are time and duration, space and externality, and similar pairs.

"Mutual externality," he declares, "is the distinguishing mark of things which occupy space." The old, time-worn disputes of philosophy concerning time, space, motion, free will, and even more recent theories that he rejects in their ordinary formulation, he endlessly reclothes in a hybrid language composed of physical, chemical, mathematical, and mechanical expressions. Thus he speaks of "fluid concepts capable of following reality in all its sinuosities," of an "ontological affinity between knower and known," of "intuition refracted into concepts and propagated to other men," of "reflective consciousness solidifying the continuous flow of reality into sensible qualities," of "Nature as a neutralized consciousness," of "the mind diluting quality into quantity," and of "reality passing from tension to extension by inversion."

The well-known assertion that accurate knowledge must lend itself to mathematical formulation is presented by him as a novel discovery, merely disguised in new language: "All the operations of intelligence tend towards geometry as their perfect achievement." He separates what belongs together—such as intelligence and instinct—in order to shift the burden of explanation for his pseudo-theories from one to the other as it suits him. He attacks Reason, Logic, and Intellect because they are too democratic, because they do not lend themselves to manipulation, and because every person can appeal to them directly and obtain redress against falsehoods imposed by philosophical charlatans. Together with other, less brilliant sophists, he attempts to restore—under the new label of Intuition—the ancient authority of revelation and inspiration:

the mystics' and spiritists' direct communion with supernatural powers, or Hartmann's Unconscious. The ordinary individual is excluded from access to such a capricious and autocratic authority and must approach it through privileged intermediaries—Bergson himself, William James, Rudolf Eucken, and their followers.

He dazzles and confuses through picturesque, wildly metaphorical, symbolic, and sonorous language.

Unlike the honest thinker, he does not employ metaphors merely as illustrations or as aids for ascending toward general concepts. Instead, he expects his metaphors to be taken literally, admired for their brilliance, but not used as instruments for independent thought. They are promissory notes that can never be redeemed for solid, nourishing facts.

He combines words denoting mutually exclusive abstract concepts, yet prudently avoids applying the same trick to concrete perceptions, knowing that those who live on the perceptual level cannot be deceived in their own domain. Thus he speaks with solemn seriousness of the "spatialization of time," the "materialization of spirit," the "concretion of durations," and "duration increasing in tension"—expressions no more meaningful than talking of painting sounds or smelling colors. In this way, he revives the primitive, anthropomorphic habit of personifying abstractions, merely dressing it in modern attire. He declares that "the universe is a great individual akin to ourselves," that "intelligence has been deposited by life on its march," that "spirit contracts into intelligence," that "by turning upon itself, the faculty of seeing becomes identified with the act of willing," that "matter is ballasted with geometry," that "intelligence insinuates itself into matter and adopts its rhythm," that "mathematics represents the direction in which matter falls back," that "physics fulfills its rôle by pushing matter toward spatiality," that "automatism lies in ambush for our freedom," and that "our activity leaps from act to act."

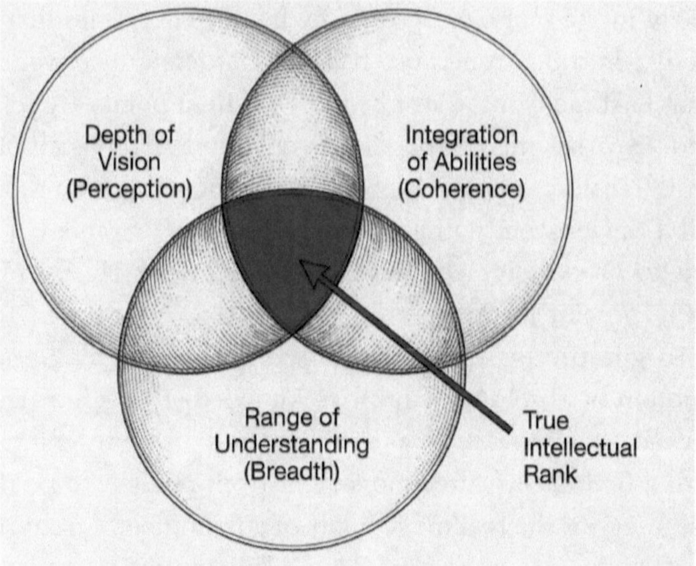

The naïve materialistic notion that ideas are mere copies or emanations of things reappears in his talk of "fluid conceptions" and of the alleged incapacity of the human intellect to grasp dynamical reality—as if the idea of motion had to move, or the idea of infinity had to be infinite. To know something, in his view, is to become identical with it, to be inside it; to perceive is to carve fragments out of a continuous stream of reality. He imagines he is doing metaphysics, while in fact he is merely rewriting physics, replacing the names of material objects with abstract terms. These confused remnants of elementary physical, chemical, and mathematical knowledge acquired at school he then serves as if they were fresh philosophical discoveries.

He avoids defining his terminology clearly, so that he may use it arbitrarily, bend it to his needs, and conceal his intellectual sleights of hand. The simple truth that nature admits of no sharp demarcation lines between phenomena is distorted into the seemingly profound doctrines of "fluid conceptions," "dilution of quality into quantity," "spatialization of time," and "concretion of durations." Yet he remains careful to behave sensibly in the realm of perception: he does not claim that Paris dissolves into Berlin because national borders are conventional, or that East melts into West because cardinal points are relative. He boldly proclaims the possibility of knowing things absolutely from the inside, yet avoids absurdity by not suggesting that we smell a flower from within it, taste an apple from its own point of view, or perceive the absolute form of a table by placing ourselves inside its drawers.

To glimpse his philosophical workshop, one may examine his notion of absolute or intuitive knowledge. It originates in a confused recollection of a simplification used in mechanics, where a fictitious relative movement from point A to point B is substituted for the real movements of a falling body from A to C and of a vehicle moving from B to C. This simplification is useful because the impact experienced would be the same in both cases. But this does not imply that the observer has no other means of knowing the real movement of the falling body than by placing himself inside it, nor does it justify transforming a practical convention into a metaphysical doctrine.

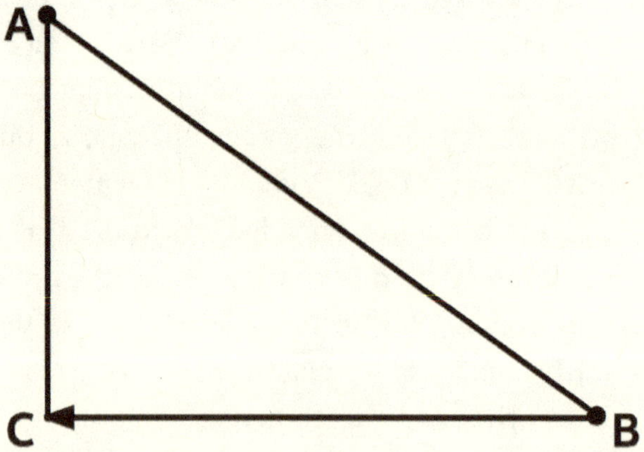

One familiar kind of senseless paradox—beloved by Bergson and by philosophical charlatans of every age—consists in seizing upon concepts that are correlated and therefore inseparable, such as space and time, change and permanence, motion (energy, force) and matter, subject (mind) and object (world), and then denying the reality of one group or reducing it to a mere derivative, shadow, or appearance of the other. These sophists are careful, however, never to apply the same procedure to correlated perceptions. They do not venture into concrete reality to tell us, for example, that the flight of birds is real while the birds themselves are fictitious, or that hunger can be satisfied by imagining food.

Just as a rapidly rotating wheel becomes impenetrable to objects thrown against it, behaving as if the spaces between its spokes were filled with matter, so a quick, sanguine, practical, restless, over-occupied, enthusiastic mind—a mind in which ideas and actions follow each other mechanically and with great speed—becomes impervious to original truths. Such a mind cannot truly assimilate or incorporate new doctrines that circulate in the intellectual atmosphere.

Spontaneity or passivity consists in the transformation of physiological energy into psychical energy. The reverse process—the transformation of conscious psychical energy into physiological energy—constitutes voluntary or active behavior. The will does not create; it merely reproduces, arranges, and directs the data supplied by spontaneity. In its earliest stage, will is self-imitation.

Personality expresses itself no less in imitation than in creation, for we cannot imitate anything that does not already exist within us at least as a tendency. The avoidance of pain and the pursuit of pleasure are the motives of voluntary action, but they are merely the results of spontaneous processes, whose causes are purely physiological—namely, a surplus of energy seeking new channels of discharge once the old channels are sufficiently supplied.

Human desires stand like gatekeepers at the entrance of consciousness. They admit only impressions that are anticipated, expected, or in harmony with them. All other impressions and memories are left outside, in the darkness of the unconscious, until by accumulation and association they gain sufficient force to break through.

In conservative, tradition-bound, letter-worshipping societies where originality and mental productivity are not tolerated, creative energy manifests itself in disguised forms: in ingenious interpretations and commentaries on traditions, ancient texts, authoritative works, and time-honored institutions. New meanings are read into old words; the unfamiliar is concealed beneath the familiar cloak of custom; expression is limited to hints, cautiously posed questions, parables, myths, and symbols.

Where intellectual energy is repressed and denied free, continuous expression as a life-calling, it erupts intermittently in flashes—proverbs, short poems, winged phrases, epigrams. Invention hides beneath imitation; hopes and ideals are presented as if they were real events of a distant past.

Inspiration and Intuition.—The cooperation of the senses and motor centers is simultaneous, instinctive, and automatic. What we hear, we tend to look at, touch, smell, act upon, or imitate, unless experience warns us otherwise. By contrast, the cooperation of higher intellectual functions—perception, memory, imagination, reasoning—is deliberate, spontaneous, irregular, and difficult to achieve.

It occurs only in certain individuals, at certain moments, and on certain topics. The accidental convergence of higher intellectual functions with emotion constitutes inspiration or intuition. If the capacities of superior individuals foreshadow the future evolution of humanity, we may hope that in a very distant future mankind will acquire the ability for constant, automatic, universal, and simultaneous cooperation of all mental functions at any moment and on any subject.

Just as social happiness will arise from instinctive and voluntary cooperation among men, and just as the highest aesthetic enjoyment would result from the harmonious cooperation of all the arts, so the highest degree of truth—almost absolute truth—will emerge from the instinctive and simultaneous cooperation of all intellectual faculties.

The lack of cooperation between sensory and motor functions is the chief source of illusion, error, and fallacy. Likewise, the absence of disinterested economic cooperation among men is the principal cause of social insecurity and misery.

The Quest of Truth.—Truth, like deep love, tolerates no rival in the heart of one who seeks it. It reveals itself only to those who renounce the pursuit of success, fame, social recognition, and wealth. The attraction of truth is so powerful for the genius that he abandons even his most cherished illusions to follow its path. For the genius, truth is an organic necessity, a permanent function; for others, it is a luxury or an occasional indulgence.

Primitive and inferior organisms cannot endure strong light; similarly, morally inferior individuals shrink from the light of truth, for it blinds the eye of their mind.

In the search for truth, we easily fall prey to prejudice—a guide that spares us effort and relieves us from the labor of seeing with our own eyes. Prejudice allows us to substitute the knowledge of classes for the knowledge of individuals, and the knowledge of the past for direct engagement with the present. Prejudices lose their inner, subjective value long before they lose their social or market value, which makes them especially difficult to eradicate.

Anticipatory attention, preconceived opinions, and prejudices can be useful if they are not relied upon excessively—if they are periodically tested, serve only to initiate thinking or overcome inertia, and never replace independent thought. The hypnotic state is marked by intense but temporary prejudices concentrated in one or a few directions, whereas the normal mental state consists of mild but persistent prejudices in many directions. Imagination and expectation both aid and obstruct perception, depending on whether they stimulate further inquiry or replace it. We often perceive things where they are not and fail to perceive them where they are, simply because our expectations do not match reality. Thus, while searching for a book in a library, we may stand directly before it and yet fail to see it because we did not expect such immediate success. In examinations, the simplest questions often appear most difficult because candidates, anticipating complexity, distrust obvious answers.

Moderate or even conciliatory statements made by declared social reformers may provoke intense hostility in the prejudiced mind, while far more radical criticisms voiced by respectable authorities are accepted indifferently or even with approval. New truths, plainly expressed by obscure, non-academic, working-class thinkers, are often ignored, belittled, or mocked by self-important and verbose authorities, who expect originality only from officially sanctioned leaders and never from below.

The broad-hearted, moral genius harbors no prejudice against human beings. Every person deserves his sympathy if worthy of it. He treats others without regard to rank or influence, guided solely by merit. He does not recoil from those deemed outcasts, but seeks the remaining kernel of goodness within them as a point of moral renewal. No individual is abandoned by him as hopeless.

Likewise, the broad-minded intellectual genius is free from prejudice toward ideas. He welcomes every thought that seeks entry into his awareness, regardless of fashion, popularity, or material gain. His chief concern is intellectual profit, which arises from the exercise of reason even when it leads to negative results. He listens patiently, and without fear of ridicule, to neglected or controversial theories, condemning none without thorough and impartial examination. Just as entrenched social leaders guard their privileges against newcomers, so do entrenched beliefs guard the gates of consciousness, excluding any facts that threaten them. The masses see only what their leaders suggest and pass blindly over whatever they have been taught to fear.

In this way, creative life, moral insight, and the pursuit of truth are bound together: all demand openness, courage, and freedom from prejudice, and all require the patient cooperation of the whole mind.

The more effort a writer expends on polishing, chiseling, and ornamenting his style, diction, and phrasing, the less genuine eagerness for truth may be expected from him. The more he seeks to please as many readers as possible—that is, the more he loves himself—the less love he places in the service of Truth. The more his attention is fixed on the impression he wishes to produce, the less it is directed toward the object of thought itself, toward the problem he claims to examine.

The genius does not require statistical masses in order to reach conclusions. A few observations—sometimes a single one—are often sufficient as the basis for far-reaching generalizations. He values a simple, precise, spontaneous, and unexpected personal observation of a phenomenon, taken together with its antecedents, accompaniments, and consequences, far more than a multitude of inaccurate, isolated, and anticipated observations gathered by others on supposedly similar phenomena torn from their natural context, or than a whole series of artificially arranged experiments.

For the same reason, the genius places little confidence in the "questionnaire" method when seeking insight into the soul and heart of his fellow men. Such a method presupposes, first, that every individual fully knows and understands himself, and second, that everyone is willing and able to give impartial and truthful accounts of his inner life. Statistical research is an excellent field for talented minds, who can verify, modify, extend, and practically apply the results achieved by geniuses. But in the flight of his imagination the genius surveys, in a single glance, a wider horizon of facts and relationships than the scientist, crawling laboriously on the surface, could explore in an entire lifetime.

Thought and Language.—Thoughts arise like plants. A certain stage of life and a certain organization of the brain are necessary conditions for their growth. Like plants, thoughts often remain for a long time in an embryonic state, hidden in the dark soil of the subconscious, before they emerge into the light of consciousness as fully formed intellectual creations.

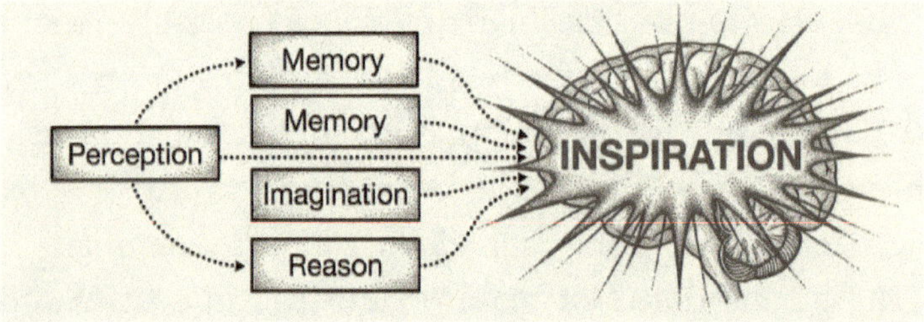

Language is never an adequate translation of thought, not even of abstract thought. There is no true parallelism between the categories and subcategories of language—its parts of speech—and those of thinking itself. Language renders only our most important, latest, and concluding states of consciousness. Superficial thinkers are therefore more talkative and more graphomaniacal—using Lombroso's expression—than profound thinkers. They reach conclusions quickly; their premises and preparatory thoughts remain incomplete; the resulting mental states are not clearly distinguished from the generating ones; genuine productive ideas are not separated from collateral or preceding states of mind; no hierarchy of value exists among their conclusions, and thus no discrimination governs which thoughts deserve expression and which do not.

Clear thinking expresses itself in clear language. The reverse is not necessarily true, but the opposite always holds: confused, mystical language does not conceal depth; it conceals confusion.

A rich vocabulary does not prevent poverty of ideas. There may be many appearances without corresponding realities, or, more precisely, different appearances may disguise the same reality rather than distinct ones, or merely different shades of a single truth. Growth in thought does not immediately entail a corresponding growth in terminology. The balanced, genuinely original mind strives, as far as possible, to work with the existing stock of words. The unbalanced inventor, by contrast, produces useless novelties: new words for old ideas, new names for slightly altered concepts, unusual word groupings to express banalities. He employs abstract and general terms to describe very concrete and particular facts. For him, the appearance of originality matters more than its reality; he hunts after appearances to deceive both others and himself about his inner sterility. To delight in such self-deception regarding declining creative power is as pathological as to indulge in unwarranted euphoria while physical health steadily deteriorates. A less distorted semi-original worries about his waning creativity, and when he resorts to verbal novelty, it is often to preserve the admiration of his followers and to prevent his name from fading from public attention.

"Ignoti nulla cupido." One who seeks originality and creation must possess, or must once have possessed, at least a germ of it; he must have tasted its pleasure. Only in the abnormal craving for originality does desire and will exceed actual capacity and physiological limits, instead of remaining adapted to them. It is not abnormal to seek consolation in appearances when reality is lost or unattainable—that is merely a sign of weakness and is common to the masses in their beliefs and customs. What is abnormal is to delight in appearance, in pseudo-originality, as though it were genuine creative power.

Between the true geniuses—original both in content and in form, in thought and in expression—and the intellectually barren philistines lies the class of semi-original individuals. Some are original in thought but not in form: their ideas remain buried in the unconscious until genuine geniuses provide them with adequate expression. Others are original only in form: they are pseudo-geniuses who dress old ideas in new language and thus appropriate the intellectual property of others by hiding it beneath a personal linguistic cloak.

We treat words much as we treat people. Some words gain popularity not because they are meaningful or useful, but because of their noble lineage—from Latin, Greek, French, or the language of a dominant class—or because of their pleasing sound or appearance. Such words are entrusted with every conceivable task; they are made to represent the most diverse ideas, even when entirely unfit for the purpose. Overburdened in this way, they end by signifying nothing at all and linger as empty sounds. Conversely, closely related functions or meanings that could be expressed by a single word are artificially separated by scholars and assigned to multiple terms, resulting not in clarity but in waste and confusion. Words equally suited to express the same idea are treated as if they conveyed different meanings merely because they sound different, while so-called noble words are elevated to privileged positions.

The genuinely superior mind, rich in real ideas, therefore uses simple, transparent, honest, and unequivocal words that faithfully convey meaning. The pseudo-superior individual, possessing few or no ideas to communicate, prefers rare, high-sounding, intoxicating, vague, aristocratic, technical, and caste-bound language, which gives only the illusion of depth, novelty, and distinction.

Just as in modern social organization much useful work remains undone while ornamental, useless, or even harmful activities are exaggerated and overproduced, so it is with language. Many valuable, beautiful, and elevating ideas, longing for expression, find no fitting linguistic form and thus remain hidden or are forced into worn-out, ambiguous garments. Meanwhile, countless trivial and meaningless ideas enjoy an abundance of elaborate linguistic costumes with which to disguise their emptiness.

Articulate language, which to the thinker is a means of imparting, acquiring, and exchanging ideas or knowledge, arouses in the mind of the philistine only confused ideas and emotions. He uses language chiefly as a channel of motor discharge: as a relief valve when he is prevented from expending his energy in the direct gratification of his needs, or as a convenient outlet for surplus energy that he does not wish to store by transforming it into sensory impressions or forces of ideas. Whoever addresses a philistine with the intention of conveying general views is therefore often painfully surprised to encounter anger, resentment, or wounded self-love. Words do not convey clear ideas to him; they merely stir feelings of attraction or repulsion, love or hatred, self-complacency or self-depreciation. He cannot conceive how anyone could speak with any intention—if with any intention at all—other than to please, flatter, court, or to irritate, insult, humiliate, or tease the listener. This explains why a speech lacking strong intonation and unaccompanied by gestures or emotional coloring fails to appeal to the masses, does not move them to action, and merely bores them. The attention of the genius resembles a finely balanced scale: the smallest weight, a fact unnoticed by ordinary minds, is enough to shift its center of gravity and set his ideas and feelings into motion. Attention is not a separate power or faculty; it is a quality of mental processes themselves—their intensity and their capacity to transmit this intensity to associated and suggested processes. The streams of consciousness flow more rapidly and are richer in content in the genius than in the average man. For this reason, it takes him so little time to bring certain thoughts into contact and to discover their connections that his reasonings often appear to others as intuitions.

Perhaps the only difference between the consciousness of the ordinary person and that of the poet or the thinker lies in its subject matter—in what it responds to and is occupied with.

And who can say whether consciousness is a purely human attribute? Do not plants and animals respond to atmospheric changes where human beings remain blind? Are not plants geniuses in nutrition, while man is often a nutritional philistine and parasite? And within our own bodies, can we deny some form of consciousness to individual cells? Do they not respond to influences that concern them alone, rather than the organism as a whole? What we call human consciousness may in fact be a higher-order consciousness, concerned with the organism taken as a whole, just as social consciousness—the state—ought to be concerned with general interests rather than with those of classes or isolated individuals. The ordinary person is chiefly conscious of daily needs; the poet is more aware of the emotional side of human experience and is often blind or tactless in practical affairs; the thinker is more conscious of the cognitive aspect and is frequently deficient in emotional and practical responsiveness.

It is probable that the cells forming an animal colony or organism possess less consciousness than independent single-celled organisms, just as individuals living in isolation, far from centers of civilization, can better appreciate the advantages of social organization than those dwelling in cities. The distribution of consciousness resembles that of static electricity in conductors:

it does not reside evenly in every particle, but accumulates on the surface and at prominent points.

The man of action, the experimenter, and the imitative artist are not fully conscious of all their aims and motives; they are chiefly aware of intended actions, immediate purposes, and the means required to achieve them. The contemplative or thinking individual, by contrast, is more conscious of ultimate aims, motives, and ends than of immediate actions and concrete means. The creative artist, the poet, and the technician are conscious of concrete particulars—individual events, details, single phenomena, or isolated states of mind. They are only dimly aware of, and express merely in hints or implicit suggestions, the classes, wholes, laws, and general ideas that rise above the limited fragment of reality forming the subject of their work. With thinkers, scientists, and philosophers the reverse is true. The philosopher, in particular, is fully conscious of general laws, comprehensive views, and broad world- and life-conceptions, which he expresses clearly and boldly, but he is less aware of, and only vaguely suggests, the countless particular cases and concrete consequences that may be subsumed under or derived from them.

Just as each cell in the organism called the human body is chiefly conscious of its own condition and immediate relations, while the brain is less aware of itself and more concerned with the general state of the whole body and with distant internal and external influences, so it is with society. The moral philistine, a mere cell of the social organism, is conscious mainly of his own needs and immediate relations. The moral genius, who functions as the brain of the social organism, is less sensitive to his own risks and sufferings and more deeply concerned with the common welfare and misery of the group, the nation, or humanity as a whole. His attention is fixed on fundamental causes and remedies of social maladjustment and human suffering. Form is at once a means of revealing and an obstacle to recognizing content, substance, and meaning; language both expresses and conceals thought.

No single form of expression can adequately convey every kind of mental content. The adequacy of a form lies in its capacity to communicate a specific state of mind. It is meaningless to call music a vague language without specifying with respect to which mental states this is true. Music is the clearest and most definite language of pure emotion; only when it attempts—such as in certain musical-dramatic excesses—to express ideas does it become vague. The same holds for articulate language: words are precise instruments for expressing ideas, but they are inadequate for conveying pure emotion and ill-suited for expressing volition. Conversely, the contents conveyed by music are vague when compared with those of articulate language. Dance, music, sculpture, painting, poetry, drama, the novel, science, and philosophy express increasingly complex states of mind, with a growing predominance of ideas over emotions and of postponed, reflective activity over impulsive action.

What applies to different modes of expression also applies within each mode. Language suitable for concrete experiences becomes misleading when used for philosophical concepts, and philosophical language obscures concrete experience. Mathematical language, perfectly suited to simple quantitative relations, becomes pedantic and inappropriate in psychology and philosophy, where we deal with qualitative and complex relations. Just as analogy can either clarify or obscure understanding—depending on whether it is used as an aid or mistaken for the reality itself—so language, form, and symbols can reveal or conceal truth, according to whether they merely stimulate attention or captivate it entirely. Form, language, symbols, customs, and rituals, so long as they remain simple and transparent, serve as vehicles for conveying meaning, thought, morality, and truth. But once they become over-elaborate, conventional, and adorned, they betray their original purpose. They absorb our attention completely and prevent us from perceiving the content they are meant to convey. We become fascinated by appearance and forget the reality behind it.

The genuinely original individual neither needs nor desires to dazzle others with pedantic, over-technical, neologistic, or figurative language. His fully developed ideas do not fear the transparency of simple, natural, commonly understood speech—just as the harmonious forms of ancient sculpture were revealed, not concealed, by simple garments.

When even honest and conscientious writers resort to ornate or fashionable expressions, they often do so under the pressure of an age devoted to word-worship and under the demands of form-loving publishers and readers. The dishonest, deliberately obscure professional writer or speaker, however, exceeds all bounds in his effort to hide falsehood, triviality, inconsistency, and intellectual emptiness behind hypnotic, ambiguous, and evasive language.

Even an intellectually honest and original thinker may fall victim to this illusion. When such a thinker mistakes verbal ingenuity for genuine originality, it is often because academic convention rewards linguistic novelty over clarity. Deception of others is inseparable from self-deception, and even great minds can be misled into confusing verbal refinement with real insight.

The use of archaic language and obsolete symbols in religious practices—forms that no longer convey clear ideas but merely arouse confused, paralyzing emotions—is commonly excused as conservatism or emotional tradition, rather than recognized as a means of psychological domination. Similarly, the use by pseudo-superior individuals of vague, technical, insinuating language, or of expressive gestures and tones no longer commonly understood, is praised as cleverness rather than exposed as cowardice, hypocrisy, or moral evasiveness.

Among modern languages, the academic use of German stands as a striking example of linguistic alienation, where the language of the educated and privileged classes diverges so far from that of the people—in grammar, sentence structure, abstraction, and complexity—that it appears to them almost as a foreign tongue.

If the poet shows a preference for archaisms, personifications, pictorial language, figures of speech, and concrete words recalling obsolete beliefs or bygone modes of life, this does not spring from intellectual dishonesty. It arises simply because the poet represents a more primitive type of thinker and therefore employs a correspondingly more primitive mode of expression.

Language is an inadequate, one-dimensional, abbreviated, selective, and merely suggestive translation of thought. It is an imperfect instrument for expressing mental life. Words may represent realities, but they may also distort them. Thus, expressions such as "saving appearances" or "diplomacy" are, in substance, identical with "lying," "intriguing," or "bluffing," yet they do not offend because they appear in a more respectable linguistic dress. Language lends an air of fixity, definiteness, maturity, and richness of meaning to what is in reality fluid, variable, dynamic, growing, many-voiced, imaginary, or even empty of content.

Not only can identical things be expressed through countless different verbal forms, but entirely opposite feelings and convictions may circulate under the same name. Hence, those who clearly perceive the absurdities and childish elements of religion, yet lack the courage to oppose the majority or offend loved ones, often abandon the substance while clinging to the name. Under the cloak of "religion" they conceal convictions that are in fact scientific, philosophical, or ethical—everything except religion itself.

Because forms are more abundant than substance, it is understandable that the same discoveries are made independently by many minds, though they rarely appear in identical linguistic forms.

Sentimental natures may grasp fragments of truth, but never truth in its completeness, because their imagination is not sufficiently guided by will and discipline. The speculative or purely subjective thinker is closer to the poet than to the thinker: he glides on the wings of imagination over the surface of things and only occasionally descends into direct contact with reality.

The greater an original mind's receptivity—that is, the more systems of ideas are disturbed and set in motion by a new thought—the more difficult initial assimilation becomes; but once harmony is achieved, it is far more stable. Those who accept foreign opinions too readily do not truly assimilate them.

Thinking and consciousness stand to emotion and unconsciousness in the same relation as the commutator of a dynamo stands to alternating currents. Spontaneous, intermittent, rhythmic emotional processes are transformed into continuous, regulated, voluntary activity. Discontinuous, exhausting effort gives way to calm, sustained volition. Painful, rare emotional shocks are replaced by steady, often even pleasurable, mental occupations.

Another essential function of thinking is the storage and regulation of volitional or motor energy. It prevents emotional and volitional forces from dissipating themselves in immediate, wasteful muscular action and preserves them as dynamic ideas until the most suitable channels for action are found. It restrains fluctuating and conflicting impulses from issuing in mutually destructive acts, holding them back until they can be harmonized and directed toward a common goal. By rehearsing action mentally—sometimes aided by small-scale experimentation—it saves the individual from irreversible consequences and needless expenditure of energy that follow impulsive, large-scale action. In this way, blind, aimless, explosive tendencies are transformed into purposeful, farsighted, economical, coordinated, regulated, constructive, and cooperative activity. It also prevents the dangerous accumulation of suppressed emotional energy that might otherwise discharge itself suddenly, violently, and harmfully. The emotional individual oscillates between opposite extremes of conduct, each undoing the effects of the other. He advances in no clear direction, reaches no lasting goal, and never stabilizes on a higher plane of life. The thinking individual, guided by reason, moves steadily toward a definite aim and toward ever wider horizons. In freeing himself from tradition, custom, routine, externally imposed obedience, and uncritical submission, he does not rush to the opposite extreme of absolute license. He does not confuse liberation from artificial, socially harmful restraints with liberation from natural, self-imposed, and socially necessary discipline. He does not pass abruptly from reverence for established doctrines to cynicism, from rigid morality to indiscriminate laxity, from blind obedience to paradox-mongering rebellion.

Unlike the purely emotional person, the thinker does not rush to destroy everything that appears obsolete or obstructive. Reason counsels him to create at least a provisional substitute before dismantling what exists.

He separates what is worth preserving from what truly deserves rejection. If he belongs to the exploited and oppressed, he does not succumb to the impulse to become an exploiter in turn. He directs his struggle against the roots and causes of oppression, not indiscriminately against individuals. He resists the temptation to free himself not only from intellectual constraints but also from moral ones, not only from drudgery but also from useful and rewarding work.

It is natural for the unthinking or intellectually intimidated individual to swing violently from one extreme to another—submission giving way to blind revolt, dogmatic faith to fanatic destruction, rigid belief to absolute skepticism—before finally settling somewhere between. The thinking person, however, performs this oscillation only in thought, not in action. By foreseeing consequences and avoiding needless reversals, he spares himself destructive experiments and advances slowly, cautiously, yet firmly along the sound and balanced middle path. The pedant dresses banalities in technical language; the popular writer, by contrast, dresses abstract and scientific ideas in the narrow idiom of the masses. The genuine man of science adapts language to thought itself. The pedant appropriates the form of culture, the popularizer appropriates its contents, but the scientist commands both.

Thinking and imagination are our mental microscope and telescope. They render the invisible and the distant visible and near, transform the past into living actuality, and turn impossibility into possibility. They extend our senses and refine our perceptions.

Art, Poetry, and Psychology

Art seeks beauty—that is, adequate, concrete, and palpable forms and symbols for thought, truth, reality, and ideas permeated with emotion, ideas that involve fundamental or higher vital interests. We need not complain that poetry has exhausted its themes. So long as the human heart and human passions remain essentially the same, no new subjects are required. Poetry's principal task is to give fitting expression to our nobler passions and longings, to discover the appropriate language and the most suitable form for humanity's vital hopes and fears. Poetry is therefore less a matter of content than of form. Form is more changeable and more fragile than essence, and for this reason poetry offers a wide field for originality.

The farther an object lies from the sphere of our senses, the weaker and less vivid its mental image becomes. Once it leaves the domain of perception and enters that of imagination, we possess no longer a presentation but only a vague representation. Since nothing can be represented that has not first been presented—since nothing can enter imagination without having once belonged to sensation—we understand why ideals can never be wholly created. They are merely new and vital combinations of representations whose corresponding sensations have already been experienced. Ideals formed in imagination react upon the sensory world and impel us to create corresponding objects in reality. Ideals are thus products of past experience and at the same time causes of future experience.

The spheres of imagination and perception, as well as those of volition or desire and power, overlap only partially. Some perceptions never reappear in imagination, and some actions that lie within our power never become objects of desire. Their common ground consists of elementary perceptions and spontaneous actions, which form the raw material for new imaginative and volitional combinations. Many of our imaginings and wishes remain forever incapable of entering the realm of perception and effective power.

Outer volition is the psychic antecedent of muscular movement; objectively speaking, it is the cerebrospinal movement immediately preceding and exciting muscular action. Thought, by contrast, is cerebral movement that is not, or only indirectly, followed by muscular activity. Abulia is therefore not, as Ribot maintains, a defect of will, but a defect of power—specifically of the muscular system. The muscles of the abulic individual, like those of a sleeping person, are too fatigued, inert, or relaxed to respond readily to volition without the aid of external stimulation.

Both poet and psychologist carry the materials of their work and their laboratory largely within their own souls. Consciousness serves them as microscope and scalpel; experimentation and observation are for them chiefly means of verification.

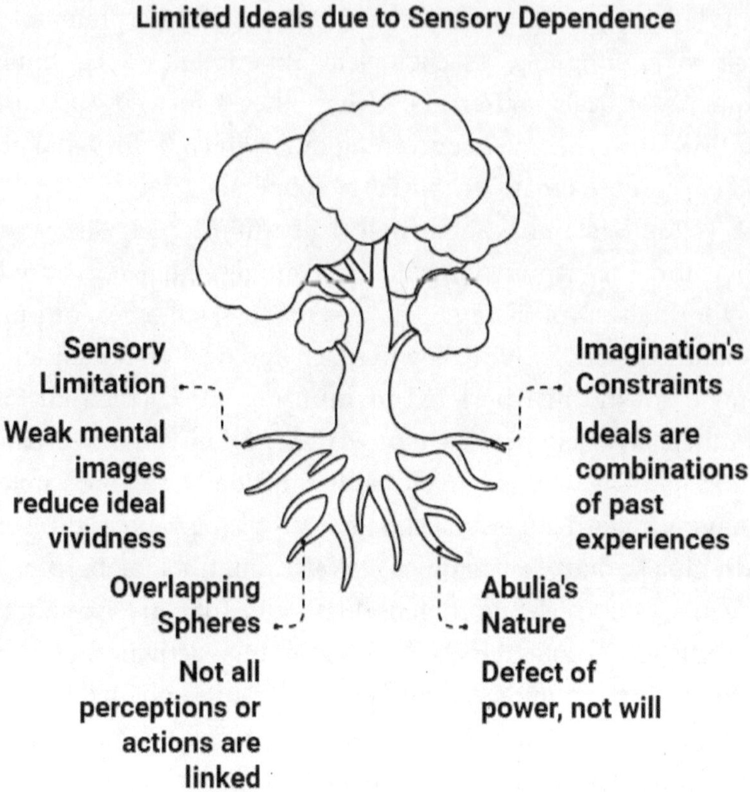

The born psychologist finds his most reliable subject of study in himself. He does not place himself or others under artificial, prearranged conditions in order to penetrate the human soul. Instead, he draws general conclusions from the daily, natural, and unsolicited experiences of life. Nor does he seek to understand others by direct questioning. He observes their actions, their outward behavior, and the unintentional revelations of character that emerge in speech and conduct when they believe themselves unobserved.

Human life, with its manifold relations and vicissitudes, provides constant shifts in perspective, external situations, and corresponding states of mind. It offers abundant opportunities to bring latent abilities to light and to uncover the most hidden corners of the soul. It continually overturns our a priori expectations about ourselves and others. Indeed, human life itself is an ongoing psychological experiment—a continuous sequence of trials and errors, of hypotheses formed, discarded, modified, or confirmed concerning our own capacities and aims and concerning others' readiness to cooperate.

To understand what people truly think, feel, desire, and strive for, the genuine psychologist judges them not by what they formally profess in books, newspapers, speeches, or public declarations, but by how they live, act, and deal with their fellow beings; not by their declared moral code, but by their customs and their privately practiced, unwritten morality; not by isolated or exceptional deeds, but by habits and daily conduct; not by behavior toward superiors, equals, patrons, or socially protected individuals, but by conduct toward inferiors, subordinates, servants, the obscure, defenseless, and dependent; not by compulsory, professional, bread-winning activities, but by spontaneous, voluntary, self-chosen pursuits; not by business friendships, but by freely chosen private friendships; not by actions performed under artificial experimental conditions, but by behavior in ordinary, natural circumstances.

The scientist and the psychologist examine and correct the simplified and idealized past of memory and imagination in the light of the present, whereas the poet strives to mold the present according to the imagined world of recollection and hope. The true poet exaggerates reality and truth not to distort them, but to throw them into sharper relief. He exaggerates accidental form in order to emphasize essence and permanence.

Only reality can normally engage our interest and sympathy—not the obvious and banal reality of daily routine, but that which is hidden, exceptional, or still ideal; the ideal striving to become real, the exceptional deserving to become the rule; the ideal constructed from realistic elements; the exceptional and even the pathological insofar as they exaggerate what is noble and valuable in human nature. For the ideal to move us, it must remain connected with real life and daily experience. Hence the naïve reader often attributes historical reality to fictional events and characters, while the more educated reader seeks at least psychological truth and plausibility.

Even readers of sensational literature are drawn to it because they believe it deals with the realm of reality and possibility. Those condemned to monotonous drudgery and deprived of opportunity, who remain ignorant of how the world is governed and how its rewards are distributed, gradually lose—if they ever possessed—the ability to distinguish wish from reality, probability from impossibility. When all near possibilities are denied them, why should they not dream of the remote or the impossible? Why should the servant girl or shop girl not dream of a prince or a hero, when even modest, attainable prospects lie beyond her reach?

Poetic description differs fundamentally from scientific description. The former is subjective, personal, and unilateral, designed to arouse emotion; the latter is objective, impersonal, and multilateral. A poetico-scientific description unites both perspectives, harmonizing subjectivity with objectivity.

The difference between the scientific psychologist and the practical knower of men—such as the diplomat, detective, or businessperson—and the difference between psychologist and poet, does not lie between analysis and synthesis. It lies between general, theoretical, explanatory knowledge and particular, practical, factual knowledge; between knowledge sought as an end in itself and knowledge used as a means. The practical observer and the poet are less concerned with why all men act or feel in a certain way than with how particular individuals or groups act and feel under specific circumstances that matter to them.

The philosophico-poetical genius breathes new life into abstract and seemingly dry thoughts. He gives spiritual values a fresh, tangible, and more attractive body—values that he himself, or an analytical thinker, has extracted from the half-prosaic flow of real life. He does not merely restore to life what has been taken from reality; he restores it on a higher and nobler plane. He revives the Past not only as it actually was, but also as it might have been, or as it was striving to become. He represents not only the Present, but also the embryonic Future contained within it—the Future that gives meaning and worth to the Present and is destined one day to replace it.

Poets, artists, novelists, technicians, and highly emotional natures may grasp fragments of general ideas, but consistent and harmonious systems of thought cannot be expected of them. At moments, they may rise to the heights of cool, abstract reflection and catch a fleeting glimpse of the subtle bonds that unite apparently disconnected situations, or of the hidden unity underlying diversity. Yet they soon lose sight of these insights when they descend again from philosophical heights into the concrete world of physical events, human actions, and passions.

The purely poetical genius is deeply impressed by events, personalities, and social conditions that are rich in ideas and ideals and that serve as vehicles of enduring truth. But he is himself unable to generalize, to separate the universal from the particular, the abstract truth from its concrete and perishable embodiment. He feels eternal truths more than he knows them. Thus, when a philosophical thinker believes he has found a kindred spirit in a poet or novelist who vividly portrays events similar to those from which he himself has derived general theories, he is often disillusioned upon closer acquaintance. He then discovers that the poet's general views—if such views exist at all—are confused and inconsistent, even with respect to the very events he renders so powerfully in art.

The pure poet or artist reproduces, with greater or lesser fidelity, what he has seen, heard, and felt, without much speculation about causes, meanings, or underlying psychological laws; without sustained reflection on what is typical, constant, and universally human, and what is merely individual, accidental, or transient. If he were as concerned as the philosopher with uncovering hidden truths and inner driving forces, he would be unable to attend to, or even remember, the small details and accessory events that give life and credibility to artistic creation.

The poet, novelist, and artist therefore stand much closer to the masses of philistines and semi-intellectual individuals than philosophers or critics usually suppose. Like the masses, they are almost exclusively interested in concrete events and unfiltered facts of daily life and struggle. They differ chiefly in emotional richness, emotional insight, and the power to synthesize and express what they see and feel. Intensified and highly differentiated emotion can even turn a philistine temporarily into a poet or novelist: it makes him notice what he usually overlooks, connect actions he normally would not relate, and step beyond his narrow personal concerns.

The pure poet, the purely emotional genius, is generally free from rigid class barriers and social prejudices. He feels at home in all social environments and participates inwardly in human dramas regardless of the stage on which they are enacted. The philosophical poet, and still more the philosophical thinker, rises above mankind itself. He frees himself from anthropocentric prejudice; his dwelling place is above the lower regions of immediate human life. He participates mentally in all that has been, is, or will be, within the infinite and eternal universe. The poet frees himself mainly from the narrow caste or social circle into which he was born; the philosopher frees himself from contemporary humanity, from the Present, even from the Earth itself.

The true poet knows how to uncover the poetry hidden in the unconscious depths of even the lowest types of men. The base aims of a criminal may still serve as instruments of the species striving toward higher ends; individual perversities may reflect submerged social ideals; hypocrisy, when expressed in more generous language, often reveals an awareness of one's own imperfections. The genuine poet also uncovers the prosaic egoism concealed behind the ostentatious altruism of pseudo-superior men. He finds enduring value in the smallest acts of the humble, detects ideal cores within perversities, and discovers a striving for harmony even within contradictory and hypocritical patterns of behavior.

Thus, behind the egotistic exploitation of the poor by capitalists, the poet may discern not only greed but also a powerful, though costly, concentration of scattered human effort—a harsh preparation for solidarity and social organization. In capitalism he sees a severe lesson, taught unconsciously by selfish individuals, revealing to society and the state what must be done to overcome misery born of uncoordinated and unsocialized labor.

The true thinker, however, is less easily dazzled by appearances or superficial imitations of truth and goodness. He detects stagnation beneath apparent progress and uncovers lingering superstition, exploitation, and parasitism hidden behind modern, flattering names. He recognizes old forms of slavery, intolerance, dogmatism, and intellectual violence persisting beneath new labels and movements, despite claims of enlightenment and reform.

Talented poets and novelists cannot easily use their present or very recent experiences as the direct material of creation. While living within these experiences, they are still actors, not yet detached observers. The reader may identify with the novel, but the writer must stand above it, possessing not only experience but also the wisdom distilled from it. The poet's present personality is a refined form of his past self. Only the humorist stands in a peculiar relation to himself: he sympathizes with his former beliefs and emotions while simultaneously ridiculing them, for he no longer shares them. When a genius seems to create directly from present experience, it is in fact older experiences, matured under the influence of the recent, that he reshapes.

The genuine creative artist selects from experience only what bears permanent human significance. This requires a broad survey of similar experiences, something possible only when they have entered memory. Immediate experience is too confused, too narrow, and too entangled with personal interests to yield general and lasting values. Memory alone is the wide and impartial repository where related experiences can gather, be compared, and purified—where beauty can be separated from ugliness, truth from illusion, and disinterested value from selfish motive.

To create is to rise high above raw experience and imagine new, harmonious combinations among elements that real life, owing to unfavorable conditions or social barriers, keeps apart. Creation brings into being ideal constellations of characters, events, and relations that would otherwise remain wasted, yet would fulfil a higher purpose if united as the creative artist envisions.

Play and Serious Activity

Play, in its narrower sense, is an abridged and softened imitation of serious activity—drawn from one's own experience, from the experience of others, from racial inheritance, or arising spontaneously. It is activity freed from harsh necessity, danger, and externally imposed aims. Play follows the direction of habit, instinct, and spontaneity.

In a broader sense, play includes children's games, leisure activities, and even art, science, and philosophy in their immature stages. Play and art begin as imitation of life but tend gradually toward transforming life according to their own ideals, becoming creative in the process. On the one hand, play refreshes us, prepares us for serious action, and reflects it; on the other hand, it creates dissatisfaction with crude reality and prepares us for a more ideal mode of existence.

The world of play, art, and imagination thus becomes both a refuge for those weary of the prosaic world and a prototype for the world that ought to be—a model of life as it might one day be transformed.

When there is a surplus of vital energy, pleasure arises from outward activity itself, regardless of how that energy is spent—whether in play or in serious action. When the amount of energy is normal, pleasure depends on the manner of expenditure, on the how—for example, in play or reverie. When energy falls below the normal level, pleasure is found not in expenditure but in restraint, in inward or intra-organic activity: rest, recovery, and recreative forms of play. If we include under the concept of play-activity every kind of activity—mental or sensory, physical or motor—that is spontaneous, involuntary, purposeless, non-oriented, self-imposed, revocable, and an end in itself, then the two classic theories of play prove inadequate. Spencer's theory, which explains play as the result of surplus energy, and Groos's theory, which views play as the expression of life-preparatory instincts, both fail to grasp its full scope. Play replaces serious or teleological activity not only when there is excess energy, but also when there is slight exhaustion or even moderate fatigue, as well as at normal energy levels—whenever external or internal pressure is relaxed, whenever urgent need or fear temporarily recedes. Children play because they are cared for; neither their own consciousness nor their guardians force them to worry about the satisfaction of vital needs. For the same reason, many women and wealthy individuals remain children throughout life, indulging continuously in bodily and mental play—sports, games, day-dreaming. Where a social class is allowed to live and thrive without effort, it inevitably drifts from purposeful, goal-directed activity into playful, aimless, undirected, automatic, capricious, and dreamy existence.

In remote prehistoric periods, when nature was generous, food abundant, and shelter unnecessary, play, reverie, and thoughtlessness were the rule, while serious activity and reflective thinking were rare exceptions. Play-activity, which puzzles the poor, the struggling, and the overburdened adult, is the natural condition of children, idlers, the wealthy, and those freed from necessity. Intellectual pursuits—artistic, scientific, philosophical, or social—appear to such minds as strange luxuries, curious forms of play requiring justification. The child takes neither bodily nor mental needs very seriously. The genius shares with the child a similar indifference toward personal material interests, and is therefore dismissed as childish by philistines and pseudo-superior men, who take such matters with exaggerated seriousness. The philistine, on the other hand, remains childish in intellectual life and is ridiculed by the genius for precisely this reason.

To call all art a form of play is to adopt the philistine's viewpoint—one that treats only material and economic pursuits as genuinely serious. To the true artist, creation is more serious, more compelling, and more irresistible than the accumulation of wealth. Artistic creation is as real a necessity as eating, drinking, or sleeping. It must be admitted, however, that the art produced for idlers, parasites, and would-be parasites—art that is shallow, ornamental, fantastic, and merely amusing—does indeed belong to the realm of play. Likewise, all arts, like all serious activities, originate in play and are indistinguishable from it in their immature stages.

Serious, realistic, thought-awakening, socially valuable art and literature are rare, because they arise from deep inner necessities. In contrast, pseudo-art and pseudo-literature—products of leisure, boredom, vanity, imitation—flood the market and shape the public's distorted view of art as mere amusement. Just as consciousness and reflection are sometimes signs of progress and sometimes of regression—useful in new and complex situations, wasteful in simple and habitual ones—so play and serious activity are not fixed opposites. At times, play signals decline from a higher, purposeful activity into aimless degeneration; at other times, it marks an advance from brutal, compulsory labor to freer, intellectual, sociable forms of action. It is likely that art began as a refined imitation of serious life—of hunting, fighting, danger, and conflict—transformed into voluntary, sociable, and leisurely expression. Early drama may have arisen from the reenactment of real disputes before the tribe: serious matters for the litigants, but instructive and entertaining for the spectators. A further step forward occurred when such representations were used not only to amuse, but to instruct, elevate, and influence the community.

Learning for immediate survival is serious activity dictated by necessity. Learning for future, possible use may appear as play from a practical standpoint, yet represents an advance when it answers a genuine intellectual need. By contrast, the amateurish engagement of the wealthy in art, philanthropy, or sentimental animal worship often reflects not progress but regression—degenerate forms of play arising from distorted serious activities.

Human development oscillates continually: from play to higher seriousness, from seriousness to higher forms of play. Theory leads to practice, practice to broader theory, and so on. To ask whether play or serious activity comes first is as futile as asking whether the hen or the egg is older. Primitive activity contains both elements without clear distinction. Instinct and intelligence, play and seriousness, action and thought are not opposites but correlated stages of one continuous process.

Wit and Humor

Wit is an intellectual play-activity. Humor stands midway between play and seriousness: playful in form, serious in intent. Serious literature presents meaning in natural, expected, transparent forms. Wit and humor, by contrast, present meaning indirectly—through disguise, incongruity, condensation, and surprise. Wit fabricates incongruities between expression and meaning, ridicules solemn matters, and plays with words and appearances. It often uses grand expressions for trivialities and trivial language for grave matters. Humor, however, uncovers real contradictions—between appearance and reality, profession and intention. It exposes sham virtue, masked vice, and undeserved seriousness. Unlike wit, humor does not spare the humorist himself.

To the witty individual, wit is an end in itself—a discharge of surplus energy or a selfish amusement. It is sometimes used by shallow writers to hide poverty of substance beneath verbal brilliance, or by cowards unwilling to express their convictions openly. Humor, by contrast, serves a moral purpose. It is one of the weapons of courage. The humorist adopts the very masks and evasions of those he criticizes in order to disarm and expose them. The philistine devotes himself wholly to bodily comfort—food, shelter, clothing. The pseudo-superior man does the same, but disguises it under the appearance of higher, altruistic pursuits. The philistine may enjoy wit and even tolerate humor, but only so long as higher aims are treated lightly, ornamentally, or indirectly. What he cannot endure is seriousness directed toward anything beyond material interest.

Thus play, seriousness, wit, humor, art, and intellect form not isolated domains, but interwoven expressions of human energy—ascending and descending stages in the long psychological movement from instinct to reason, from necessity to freedom, and from mere existence toward meaning.

The philistine may enjoy wit and even tolerate humor, but he has no understanding of the serious thinker who goes straight to the core of a problem, both in thought and in expression. Serious intellectual pursuits demand far more energy, courage, and independence than even the materially successful philistine—selected and preserved by our system of spoliation—can usually command. His critical judgment and spontaneity have been crushed by exploitation; his energy is absorbed by drudgery or uncertainty, wasted on artificial needs and ridiculous fashions imposed by shrewd commercialism, and diverted by the example of parasitical aristocracies into insatiable, degenerative, and antisocial pursuits of luxury, wealth, and empty distinctions.

The humoristic writer spares his readers mental labor by caricaturing reality. He exaggerates, highlights, personifies, and visualizes its hidden or vitally important traits, while suppressing, simplifying, or distorting others, in order to irresistibly draw attention to what truly matters. The serious thinker, by contrast, strives to depict reality in its complexity and to assign due weight to all its elements. He therefore fails to appeal to the masses, who are unable to concentrate on more than one object at a time or to grasp subtle, remote, and mediated relations—especially those that lie hidden beneath appearances and connect entire classes of phenomena.

Dream and Dramatic Activity

In reverie or daydreaming, trains of ideas and feelings that have been rejected or suppressed during purposive, goal-directed thinking rise spontaneously into consciousness. There are two principal forms of reverie:

1. Reverie as a reaction to mental exhaustion following fruitless teleological effort.
2. Reverie arising from a surplus of mental energy left after the immediate needs of life have been satisfied.

The chief difference between daydreaming and night-dreaming lies in coherence and awareness. In night dreams, purposeless and suppressed idea-trains easily displace one another, obscuring and fragmenting meaning. In daydreaming, the imagined drama is often pursued into the smallest and most trivial details.

Another difference lies in awareness of unreality: in daydreams we usually retain a dim or clear sense that what we imagine is not real; in night dreams, imaginations are mistaken for realities. This occurs because clear sensory impressions are absent—impressions that would otherwise allow us to recognize our images as mere copies or distorted combinations of past experience. It is natural to mistake imitations for originals when no direct perception corrects them.

Dreams are often translations of bodily, organic, or coenesthetic sensations into psychical imagery. We do not become directly conscious of these bodily states; we encounter them only as the emotional core or outcome of dream-dramas improvised from habitual hopes and fears.

The difference between the reverie of the ordinary person and the dramatic imagination of the novelist, poet, or artist lies in scope and value. In reverie, the dreamer's own ego is the central figure, and personal wishes, hopes, and fears form the substance of the drama. True drama, however, transcends the individual ego and addresses interests that are general, enduring, and socially significant.

Dream Activity

Between waking consciousness and dreamless sleep lies an infinite gradation of mental states, ranging from the highest coherence and rationality to extreme incoherence and meaninglessness. For this reason, it is nearly impossible to draw a sharp boundary between dreaming and waking thought. Compared with waking thought, dream activity is distinguished mainly by the absence of control by sense impressions. Dreams draw their material from memory—stored impressions—though their starting point may be an isolated bodily or peripheral sensation. Dreams usually do not culminate in motor action, except in cases such as somnambulism.

Those awakened during dreams occurring long after falling asleep or long before natural waking are especially struck by their incoherence and irrationality. The governing law of dream activity is cerebral fatigue. Brain centers that have been most used and most fatigued fall asleep first; those most easily restored resume activity first. Hence, dreams revive pictorial thinking, long-forgotten individuals, remote incidents, and even ancestral traces. Sensory and motor impressions are weakest in dreams because the sense organs and muscular system are the most exhausted and overworked parts of the organism. Isolated sensations, lacking corroboration from other senses, are therefore misinterpreted or exaggerated, producing illusions and hallucinations. Associated sensations yield perception; isolated ones yield illusion.

Despite his ingenious diagnostic use of dreams, Freud's interpretation of dreams as disguised fulfillments of repressed wishes is one-sided and incomplete. Dreams realize not only wishes, but also fears and apprehensions. Attempts to reduce such fears to early childhood wishes do not accord with reality. A student does not wish to fail an examination, nor an actor to miss the performance—yet both often dream of such events. The incoherent, pictorial, primitive quality of dream thought is better explained by cerebral fatigue than by wish-fulfillment alone.

Fatigue affects mental functions in proportion to the work performed and the available energy of each cerebral organ. Both the oldest and the most recently developed centers—perceptual and conceptual—are most vulnerable. During sleep, perceptual and motor centers are exhausted from overuse; reasoning centers from insufficient energy. Dream material therefore consists largely of images and memories mistaken for realities in the absence of perceptual correction. We dream less of what occupies us intensely during the day and more of what has receded from conscious attention.

Primitive forms of thinking, feeling, and acting reappear in dreams because recently acquired inhibitory and purposive capacities are temporarily inactive. In such states, distinctions between wish and fact, belief and knowledge, intention and ability dissolve.

Philosophy, Science, and Ultimate Concepts

From the heights of philosophical abstraction, the concrete world of objects, animals, and men may appear so distant and dim that some philosophers—idealists and solipsists—are tempted to deny its existence altogether, reducing it to a mere complex of ideas. Were these thinkers not compelled to descend from abstraction to satisfy bodily needs, some would deny the world not only in theory but also in practice, as certain forms of mental pathology demonstrate.

Idealism overlooks a crucial fact: imagination cannot create new elements or attributes; it can only recombine what experience has already provided. The question remains unanswered: why do we attribute externality and spatial reality to some states of consciousness and not to others? Because hallucinations sometimes produce the experience of external objects where none exist, some philosophers infer that even normal perception might be a kind of hallucination—a purely mental construction. Such conclusions arise not from a sober examination of experience, but from losing sight of the concrete world while gazing too long at the abstractions of thought.

Leaving aside the absurdity into which the idealistic doubt would drive us—namely, speaking of an internal world while simultaneously denying the external world, as if the term "internal" had any meaning without reference to the "external," to which it is inseparably correlated—let us put this logical contradiction aside and raise a psychological objection instead.

Even if what we take to be external objects could sometimes be unmasked as internal, subjective constructions, the reverse never occurs. No being that we initially know as a purely imaginary creation later proves itself to be a real object of the external world. The external world gives rise to our internal representations; but the internal world never introduces new elements into external reality, nor does it build real complexes out of purely imaginary constituents.

Scientific Laws

Scientific laws are said to express constant relations between phenomena and to demonstrate the uniformity of Nature. What we often forget is that what appears approximately constant to us may be highly variable to beings endowed with a more refined mathematical or perceptual sense—beings for whom an error of one-millionth of a millimeter or of a second would be significant. What we call equilibrium may in reality be a rapid succession of imperceptible oscillations in opposite directions, since even the smallest environment is never absolutely homogeneous. One would smile at a savage who, unable to conceive numbers beyond ten, formulated a scientific law declaring that never more than ten immigrants could arrive together on his island.

Men rarely suspect how little absolute uniformity, constancy, or strict periodicity exists in Nature. Just as the ordinary citizen remains unaware of the extent of arbitrariness, conflict, favoritism, and insecurity within governmental institutions, so the layman remains ignorant of the uncertainty and disagreement that pervade science and philosophy. He projects his own mental inertia—his conservatism, monotony, and desire for stability—onto Nature and onto his rulers. Nature appears constant, and authority appears secure, only so long as he remains within the narrow sphere of his immediate practical interests. Theories seem reliable because, in practice, no one relies on them alone; just as men trust one another only insofar as they are not wholly dependent upon one another.

Causation

Our belief in the constancy of Nature is largely an effect of psychical inertia—the tendency of the mind to persist in established modes of thought and to resist change. In past experience, a visible and easily accessible quality A has been associated with an invisible and less accessible quality B. When A appears again, we naturally expect B to follow. If later experience presents A without B, we initially resist this dissociation; only gradually does the old association weaken. Sometimes, instead of questioning the association itself, we question whether the newly observed A is truly identical with the former A.

What holds in perception holds equally in conceptual thought. The conviction that identical causes produce identical effects—without excluding the possibility that practically identical effects may arise from practically dissimilar causes—is itself a product of psychical inertia applied to the totality of experience. It is strengthened by our capacity to predict future events on the basis of past ones.

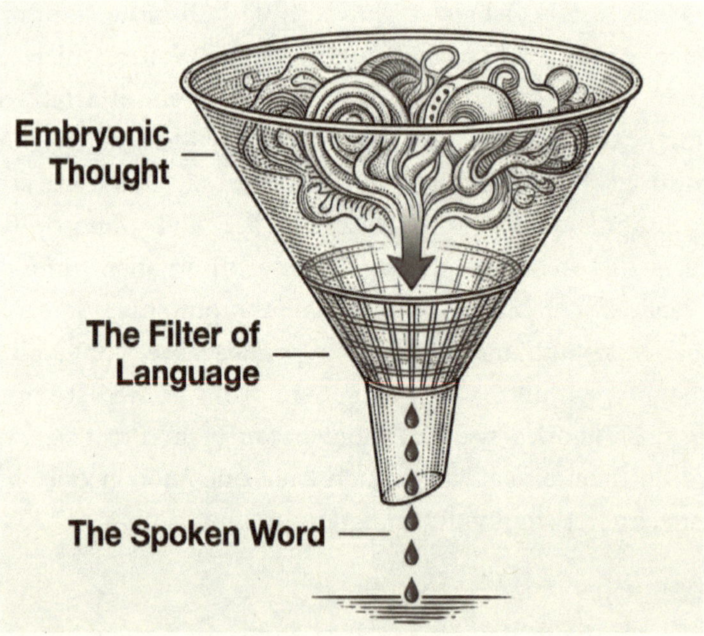

To the objection that, owing to the perpetual flux of reality, no identical causes or events can ever recur, the answer is simple. When we speak of identity, we mean identity as it appears to us. If our imperfect senses cannot detect slight variations in causes, they will likewise fail to detect corresponding differences in effects. This practical identity is sufficient for human foresight. We are concerned not with how things might appear to hypothetical superior minds, nor with "things-in-themselves," but with how they affect our actual human senses.

What distinguishes mind from matter is that, in mental life, effects may precede causes, whereas in the physical world causes precede effects. In consciousness, the effects and causes of activity are identical in essence and differ only in form. Sensations and ideas that arise unintentionally as pleasurable effects may later reappear as representations that become the causes or aims of renewed activity.

Bergson describes psychical causation as circular, in contrast to physical causation, which he calls rectilinear. It seems more accurate to describe psychical causation as spiral: a circle would allow no room for development or variation, whereas a spiral implies repetition with advance.

In the physical world, causes and effects must likewise be identical in essence or quantity, if we accept that motion can only be transferred, increased, or diminished, never created anew—just as matter cannot create matter. When it appears that identical effects arise from dissimilar causes, this is usually an illusion caused by our failure to disentangle true causes from irrelevant circumstances, by confusing partial with total causes, or by overlooking the prior activity of the reacting body itself. Alternatively, dissimilar causes may share a single common property responsible for the similar effect, while their differing properties play no role in the outcome.

Laughter illustrates this clearly. It is a mistake to treat laughter as a single effect arising from unrelated causes. Physiological laughter differs fundamentally from psychical laughter, and the latter varies according to whether it expresses genuine joy, irony, hostility, hypocrisy, or envy. As a complex phenomenon, laughter arises from a complex of causes. What all forms of laughter share, however, is one partial cause: an incongruity between appearance and reality, between the actual and the ideal, between intention and achievement—an incongruity that stimulates our self-feeling. Philosophically, unlike causes cannot yield like effects; practically, however, they may sometimes be treated as such.

If we assume that all phenomena ultimately reduce to transfers and transformations of movement; that motion is the primordial state of matter and rest merely suspended motion produced by opposing forces—we can understand how effects may appear as genuinely new creations, differing in quality and quantity from their causes, while still containing no more and no less potential matter or motion than those causes. This explains how poisonous substances may yield harmless products, how light added to light may result in darkness, and why children of the same parents, or even unrelated individuals, may differ so profoundly in actual life while remaining potentially similar.

To solve the mystery of the origin of organic life would be to explain how rectilinear, inorganic causation transformed itself into circular—and ultimately spiral—causation.

Acquisition and Limits of Human Knowledge

The average man seeks pleasure and satisfaction; the genius seeks truth. Because pleasure is more easily and directly attained through instinctive, habitual, and imitative activity, whereas truth is a contingent and often accidental outcome of spontaneous inquiry, the life of the average man tends to move in circles, endlessly repeating itself. The life of the genius, by contrast, moves in a spiral—never wholly repeating itself, always advancing, even when it seems to return to familiar ground. In this difference lies both the limitation of common knowledge and the promise of human progress.

Philosophers who adhere rigidly to a system of their own—or to one they have adopted—are usually blind to new facts that do not fit within its framework. Often they refuse to yield even to compelling evidence. Much as political parties differ loudly in theory yet act similarly in practice, philosophical systems and philosophers frequently differ more in labels, terminology, stylistic preferences, and a few paradoxical assertions than in their fundamental ideas and outlooks. Philosophers without a fixed system, or those whose systems remain flexible, are generally more open-minded and more receptive. The common individual, by contrast, readily accepts even absurdities and impossible relations, especially when these flatter personal desires, fears, or hopes. Superstition thus appears at both extremes of the human hierarchy: negative superstition at the top, and positive superstition at the bottom.

Abstract reasoning is almost absent in higher animals and remains weak even in many human beings. It may therefore be regarded as a relatively late acquisition in the evolution of our species. Whether humanity, in its future development, will acquire entirely new and higher capacities, or will merely refine those it already possesses, remains an open question.

Human knowledge begins in darkness—ignorance of the elements—and ends in confusion when faced with their more complex combinations and interrelations. There is darkness both within and beyond the sphere of human understanding. A philosophy that proceeds synthetically upward from supposed elements has no decisive advantage over one that works analytically downward from complex phenomena; both begin and end in uncertainty and perplexity.

The macrocosm and the microcosm—the infinitely large and the infinitely small, the beginning and the end of things, the primary cause and the ultimate goal of events—remain hidden from view and will likely remain forever beyond the reach of human comprehension. Perhaps this is because they possess no absolute, objective existence. What is imperceptibly small and simple for us, forming a microcosm, might be perceptible and overwhelmingly vast to a hypothetical thinking microbe, for whom it would constitute the universe itself.

The farther we attempt to trace an event or process—whether forward toward its effects and future consequences, or backward toward its causes and origins; whether by synthesis or analysis, induction or deduction; whether toward ever larger wholes or ever smaller constituents—the deeper grows the darkness that envelops our limited intellect. The experiences of single individuals, or even of a few generations, become increasingly unreliable as guides. To attempt an indefinite reconstruction of past or future events based on a narrow range of known facts is an undertaking that exceeds genuine human capacity. Yet the failure of such attempts does not prove their eternal futility, nor does it justify theological surrender. As Diderot observed, if the light of our intellect resembles a candle illuminating only a tiny portion of the path, this is no reason to extinguish it and grope blindly in the dark, guided solely by faith compounded of fear, hope, unrealizable wishes, and unfounded anxieties. How can we demand certainty about the past or future when we scarcely understand the present? If we are barely conscious of what directly affects our senses, how can we expect science to yield unquestionable knowledge of phenomena that do not act upon them at all, or only indirectly?

The ordinary individual acquires knowledge chiefly from without; in the genius, knowledge unfolds from within; in the superior individual of great talent, both processes advance toward one another, as in the tunneling of a mountain. This convergence explains the greater speed and success with which the gifted individual acquires understanding.

Knowledge gained through inner development and knowledge received verbally from others differ so profoundly in form that the genius often fails to recognize them as referring to the same object. He may believe himself to possess two distinct insights where in reality there is only one, and thus fail to recognize his own ideas in the expressions of others. This resembles the phenomenon of internal autoscopy described by Dr. Sollier, in which patients cannot identify visceral sensations with the verbal knowledge they possess of the same organs. A similar difficulty occurs in individuals who regain sight after blindness: at first, they experience visual objects as entirely new and unrelated to those previously known through touch.

Every classification of the sciences presupposes a philosophical system that serves as its perspective. Change the system—or the vantage point—and the arrangement of sciences changes accordingly. What appears coordinate, subordinate, or superordinate from one perspective may not appear so from another. The ideal perspective would be one situated at infinity, from which only a single classification would be possible—or perhaps none would be required at all.

Pseudo-superior individuals guard jealously the artificial boundaries between nations and between sciences. They forget that no advanced science, like no civilized nation, can remain self-sufficient. Progress demands cooperation and division of labor. Each science must concentrate on the tasks it can perform most effectively, drawing upon the methods and results of others and offering its own contributions in return. Just as modern workers are beginning to recognize that they share more interests with workers of other nations than with the ruling classes of their own, so too certain bodies of knowledge traditionally assigned to one science may find deeper affinities with those of another.

Facts and Hypotheses

Hypotheses are intended to explain what is distant, past, future, complex, unknown, or imperceptible—the microcosm—

by means of what is near, present, simple, familiar, and perceptible—the macrocosm. Does this not imply that truth already exists within us in germ, that it need not be created but merely uncovered and unfolded? Is it not strange to elevate our inability to transcend the data of our senses into a supposed law of nature or necessity of logic?

The development of hypotheses, theories, and philosophical systems may be represented schematically. In the first, or rectilinear stage, a hypothesis explains only a few isolated facts. In the second, or circular stage, it becomes broader and more inclusive, accounting for additional facts and relations. In the third stage, the movement continues toward greater comprehensiveness and refinement, approaching a more flexible and living understanding—one that does not close itself within rigid boundaries, but remains open to correction, expansion, and growth.

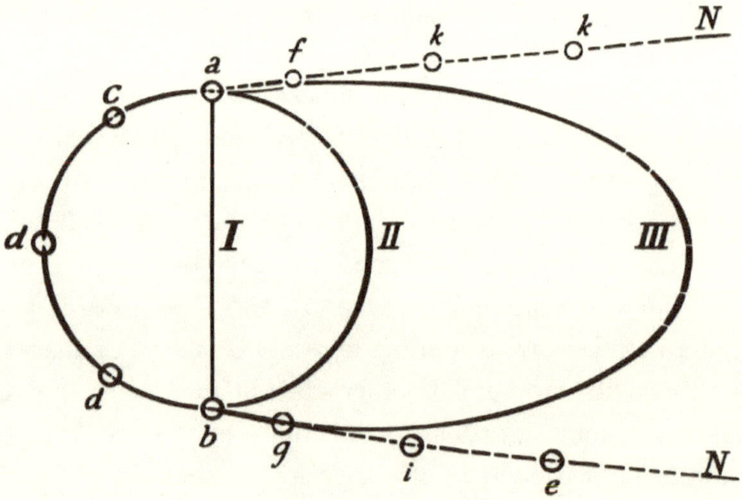

Thus, human knowledge does not advance by final answers or immutable systems, but by a continual, living movement—one that accepts uncertainty without surrendering inquiry, and that progresses not in closed circles, but along an ever-widening spiral.

1. Stages in the Growth of Theories

1. The first, or rectilinear stage, explains or connects only a few isolated facts: a, b.
2. The second, or circular stage, is broader and more inclusive: it explains additional facts or systems of facts: c, d, e.
3. The third, or elliptical stage, and
4. The fourth, or parabolical stage, extend still further in scope and inclusiveness.

For a theory to be genuinely supported, the facts invoked in its favor must be inexplicable by any other theory. Facts are the raw material—the bricks or stones; hypotheses and theories are the cement and mortar. Both are means for erecting spiritual edifices that give meaning and delight to the human mind. A purely speculative system resembles a structure made only of mortar; a purely experimental system—if such were even possible—resembles a pile of stones without binding material. Both are unstable and liable to collapse.

It has always seemed strangely comical to hear experimenters, observers, scientists, and even philosophers insist solemnly that they wish to remain strictly within the domain of facts and science, and that they refuse to venture into hypotheses, speculation, or metaphysics. In reality, every fact, every experiment, and every science rests upon some theory or metaphysical assumption and inevitably leads to broader and bolder speculation. We never perceive things and their connections exactly as they are; we perceive them largely as we imagine them to be.

The difference between so-called matter-of-fact thinkers and speculative thinkers is not that the former dispense with theories, but that they employ them unconsciously and implicitly. They are unable to distinguish fact from theory, physics from metaphysics, and they cannot rise from a limited set of observations to a wider class of facts or to a more comprehensive explanation. Speculative thinkers, by contrast, use hypotheses consciously and explicitly, and are capable of advancing toward ever higher standpoints and ever broader perspectives.

It is equally amusing to hear academic philosophers of various idealistic schools maintain that ideas, feelings, or the mind alone are real facts, while objects, the external world, and matter are mere hypotheses, non-existent, or forever unknowable. If objects do not exist, why can no idealist formulate even a single statement purely in terms of ideas without implicitly referring to objects? If objects are entirely beyond our reach, how did we come to speak about them at all?

The same contradiction appears among those who claim that energy, force, movement, or change alone is real, while matter and permanence are mere appearances or mental constructs. If this were true, why can such dynamists or energists not utter a single statement without invoking matter? Those who reduce matter to energy, electricity, electrons, or a hypothetical ether imagine they have destroyed the concept of matter, yet fail to see that ether or energy now plays exactly the role matter once played for materialists. These learned individuals, who would doubt the sanity of anyone unable to grasp why a sentence requires both subject and predicate, fail to recognize the absurdity of asserting movement without moving things, or perception without anything perceived.

Progress in Knowledge and Understanding

Since there are no absolutely isolated objects and no absolutely isolated states of mind, all knowledge is necessarily comparative, relative, and dynamic. This does not mean that we know only relations and changes. We cannot know change without some awareness of the preceding state, nor can we know relations without some knowledge of the related things themselves. We cannot know the self without knowing other selves and the external world with which it stands in constant interaction.

Just as reaction has no meaning apart from action, knowledge of things—their action upon the mind—goes hand in hand with knowledge of our own mental reactions. Things cannot be known apart from their relations, because things are nothing but centers where relations converge and condense, much as nerve cells are junction points of nerve fibers. The distinction between thing and relation is therefore one of degree and complexity, not of kind.

Knowledge is the collective name for sensing, perceiving, conceiving, and being conscious. Understanding is a higher, deeper, more comprehensive form of knowledge—conceptual, causal, and penetrating. To know a thing is to compare it, to relate it to others and to ourselves, which necessarily involves abstraction from some relations in favor of others. The same object impresses us differently depending on the standpoint from which it is viewed. Thus, the same kind of work may appear tedious or pleasant, endless or fleeting, depending on whether attention is focused on the whole or on its parts, on the goal or on the means, on one task alone or on many competing concerns. To speak of knowing "things-in-themselves" is to speak of knowing things that do not act upon the mind—no less absurd than speaking of seeing objects that do not affect the eyes or hearing sounds that never reach the ears. Likewise, to know the mind-in-itself would mean to be conscious of a mind that neither acts nor reacts, which is a contradiction in terms.

To say that reaction is equal to action is to deny spontaneity and self-activity. Even to say that total reaction equals total action remains unsatisfactory, for it implies that everything derives its entire being from external influences alone, rendering matter naturally inert—a conception that creates more difficulties than it resolves. It is more accurate to say that reaction is proportional to action. If consciousness is the total reaction of the mind to external influences, then different degrees of knowledge of the same object arise from differences in the internal conditions and activity of the mind. When too many impressions act simultaneously, or when one acts with overwhelming force, the mind can no longer respond as a whole; it fragments, lapsing into sub-consciousness or confusion. The mind can perceive only successively. To gain breadth and simultaneity, it must sacrifice clarity and deal in symbols rather than in direct realities.

Consciousness of objects and self-consciousness are two inseparable aspects of a single process. From this parallelism it follows that it is erroneous to claim we understand mind better than matter, or matter better than mind. We are equally limited—and equally informed—about both. We understand others, society, and the world only to the extent that we understand ourselves.

If our knowledge of the body and of the external world comes through identically constituted nerves, and if self-knowledge develops alongside knowledge of the not-self, then causality cannot be merely a subjective notion abstracted from voluntary action and projected outward. Were causality merely subjective, humanity would eventually abandon it, as it has abandoned animism. Instead, its hold on human reasoning has grown stronger. Causality is nothing more than a concise name for the mutual influences between things—a reality no sane observer denies.

The advance of psychology has always paralleled the advance of our understanding of the external world, though not at the same pace. Internal relations regulate themselves automatically, while external relations require conscious effort.

Hence, humans have historically devoted more attention to external facts than to inner processes. In ancient times, when survival depended chiefly on struggles against nature and rival tribes, external knowledge was paramount. In modern individualistic societies, where struggle is largely social and interpersonal, knowledge of the mind has become increasingly important. The average villager resembles a naturalist; the average city-dweller, a psychologist—though often one with knowledge but little true understanding.

Thus, human knowledge does not progress toward absolute certainty, but toward ever-broader, more flexible comprehension. It advances not by denying speculation, but by refining it—by binding facts and hypotheses together into structures that remain open, revisable, and alive.

Our body is just as external to consciousness as the surrounding physical world. For this reason, the way we come to know our own body does not differ in principle from the way we come to know the external world; neither kind of knowledge can be regarded as more objective or more certain than the other. The reason we know, from direct sources, less about the processes taking place within our own body than about external phenomena lies in the nature of these processes themselves. Inner organic processes are constant, regular, rhythmic, and uniform, whereas external phenomena are irregular, continuously changing, and lack any rhythm that is immediately perceptible (though not inconceivable). The inner, organic nerves do not differ in their structure from the peripheral, outer nerves.

Our knowledge of other minds is just as inferential as our knowledge of any material object that does not impress all our senses, such as distant stars, or that does not impress them directly, such as electrical or magnetic phenomena. If the cerebro-molecular movements of others could directly affect our highest, synthetic brain centers—rather than reaching us through their coarse and superficial muscular expressions—we would know other minds just as much, or just as little, as we know our own.

As our powers of observation and voluntary attention increase, we become aware of ever finer differences between the behavior of inanimate objects, other human beings, and ourselves. In doing so, we gradually free ourselves from animism—from the tendency to personify matter, especially moving objects, and from the habit of projecting our own thoughts, feelings, and intentions behind the actions of others. For however similar the outward actions of different people may appear, they always differ in their inner and less obvious aspects so long as they arise from different psychological causes.

It may even be that our powers of observation are not inherently greater than those of primitive peoples. Rather, we notice better than they did the less striking and less immediately useful aspects of reality—the configuration of wholes—because the knowledge of what is striking and practically useful has already been transmitted to us or made easier to acquire. Our attention is no longer monopolized by bare necessities, leaving a surplus of intellectual energy for more general, refined, and theoretical insight.

The philistine remains ignorant of himself because his development comes to an early halt. There is little change or variety in his pursuits, thoughts, or feelings; he differs neither from his neighbors nor from himself at different stages of life. The superior man, by contrast, is driven to self-analysis by the continual widening of his intellectual horizon and by the painful awareness of his difference from others—an awareness reinforced through repeated disappointments, misunderstandings, and mistreatment by philistines, and especially by pseudo- or parasitical superior men whom he has mistakenly taken for his equals. Sensation, perception, memory, imagination, judgment, and reason are not independent receptacles or grinding machines that exist apart from the material they process. In the living mind, functions and experiences are interdependent and mutually determining. Only those external vibrations for which the brain possesses corresponding, sympathetically vibrating centers can give rise to definite sensations and perceptions. In the absence of such centers, there is no clear experience—only a shock, often destructive to nerve tissue. Thus, because the human brain lacks centers that vibrate sympathetically with electrical waves, it cannot respond to them adequately or safely; many microorganisms perish under light waves because they lack optical sensitivity. If intense electrical discharges like lightning were a constant feature of the environment, humanity could not survive unless it developed brain centers capable of responding sympathetically to them.

A similar principle operates in social life. Individuals—such as the genius or the insane—who cannot vibrate sympathetically with their surroundings, who cannot imitate their neighbors to some degree, are not tolerated and are often persecuted, especially in compact, primitive communities where constant mutual observation prevails. The unspoken law is: imitate or perish. If society possessed genuinely philanthropic institutions that vibrated sympathetically with criminal or extra-social elements, it would be less endangered by them. The moral genius is precisely one whose brain vibrates sympathetically with the exploited, the disinherited, and the ill-treated, and whose intelligence is pressed into the service of this altruistic sensitivity. No amount of intellect can enable the wealthy egoist to grasp the cruelty of a system of exploitation, because he lacks sympathetic feeling for the exploited.

Somnambulists, hypnotized persons, fanatics, and individuals with rigid, one-sided opinions—those in whom certain ideas are excessively active—are blind to everything except what resonates with their dominant mental state. During an individual lifetime, very few new brain centers are formed; most are hereditarily predetermined. Because of these inherited predispositions—shaped in turn by the frequency and intensity of ancestral stimuli—we attend more readily to living beings than to inanimate objects, to animals more than plants, to movement more than rest, to human beings more than animals, and to matters directly affecting our well-being more than those of indirect relevance.

Hereditary predispositions and the intensity or frequency of personal experience determine the adequacy and reach of mental reactions. The same experience may remain, in some individuals, at the level of raw sensation; in others, memory centers are activated and sensation becomes perception; in still others, higher synthetic centers are engaged, transforming perception into apperception. In imaginative individuals, memories arise spontaneously and establish new connections, enriching the mental field still further.

Intelligence, or mental adaptability—the capacity to acquire new experiences, act upon them, relate them to past experiences, and synthesize them into classes—is not a single, uniform ability. It is a collection of partial capacities, dependent on inherited interests and external opportunities. A person may be highly intelligent in one domain and remarkably obtuse in others. A passionate individual may display ingenuity in gratifying a passion yet remain blind to the overall harm it causes. A commercial philistine may be clever in profit-seeking yet reveal profound stupidity when applying the same logic to religion or higher pursuits, judging them solely by safety or advantage. Much of the credulity seen in children and even in otherwise intelligent adults stems simply from lack of experience. Every complete perception presupposes the cooperation of memory, imagination, judgment, and reason. Yet beyond a certain point these functions cease to cooperate equally. In some individuals observation predominates; in others, memory or imagination; in still others, abstract reasoning. Thus, minds differ not only in the material they engage with, but also in the dominant mental function—observers, artists, poets, thinkers. In modern usage, intelligence often means skill in understanding people, for in a technically advanced yet parasitical society many urban dwellers live by their wits—their ability to influence, please, and manipulate others.

Evolution of Knowledge

When an object first impresses the mind of an infant, it likely produces a vague, undifferentiated cluster of sensations in which accidental and essential qualities are equally obscure. When the same object appears again, its permanent qualities are perceived more clearly than its accidental ones, because the former reinforce previous impressions while the latter vary with circumstances. To perceive an object, therefore, is to notice what remains constant across repeated experiences. Likewise, when several objects of the same class are presented, what they share in common is grasped more readily than what distinguishes them individually, because the common features are repeated and reinforced. Class attributes are thus apprehended before, or more clearly than, individual attributes.

To conceive is to notice what is common to many objects coexisting in space. To form higher-order concepts is to notice what is common to related concepts of a lower order. In this way, knowledge ascends from sensation to perception, from perception to conception, and from conception to ever more comprehensive understanding—not by abandoning experience, but by refining and organizing it into progressively broader and more coherent forms.

If the knowledge of perceptible class qualities precedes the knowledge of individual qualities, the reverse is true for the knowledge of individuals and groups. At first, all individuals belonging to the same class are mistaken for one and the same being, or for identical individuals. Only later are these individuals distinguished from one another, and with this differentiation the correlated notions of individual and class, part and whole, are gradually acquired. In the beginning, we distinguish only those groups that differ from each other in a striking, obvious manner and that are mutually exclusive; later, we learn to discriminate between classes that are closer to one another and that include or overlap each other. The scientific or logical hierarchy of classes does not, of course, run parallel to the psychological or common-sense classifications, whose divisions rest mainly on superficial and immediately perceptible qualities.

What has been said about the origin and development of objective knowledge applies, with appropriate modifications, to subjective or introspective knowledge as well. When we begin to attend not merely to the content of our mental processes, but also to their form—not only to the what, but to the how of our experiencing, feeling, and reacting—we discover that something constant recurs in the manner of our awareness. This constant element is independent of, and prior to, the particular causes or materials of cognition, feeling, or volition. This enduring form, this channel in which our streams of experience flow and to which they must adapt themselves, we call the self, the ego, character, temperament, or individuality.

Like the bed of a river, the self is, on the one hand, pre-existent to particular experiences, and, on the other, it is deepened, broadened, and sometimes even redirected by early experiences. Once formed, however, the self exerts a shaping and guiding influence on later experiences. The genius, as distinguished from the average person, possesses a self that is more or less fully developed from the beginning, and therefore molds, selects, and directs experience rather than being shaped by it. The self of the genius is active from the outset; that of the common person is passive in early life with regard to suggestion and education, and becomes active only later. The self of the average individual is teachable and largely the product of intentional and unintentional social influences; the self of the genius is unteachable and becomes, instead, a source of change in human attitudes.

There is no greater mystery in understanding the identity of the self than there is in understanding the identity of the not-self, the objective world. If the external world—and our own body may be regarded as part of it—supplies the material of our mental life, while the mind provides the form, then amidst the changing contents and changing forms of our thoughts there remains something constant, something ever recurring. This constitutes the two interacting principles we call self and not-self, mind and cosmos.

What logic treats as an ultimate concept or category of thought is, psychologically, primary and given at first in the form of vague, meaningless sensations. What logic regards as last is first for psychology. This gradual progression from obscure sensation to meaningful interpretation can be clearly observed when attention is distracted during or after an experience. If the mind is absorbed elsewhere when an internal or external stimulus occurs, we are at first merely aware that something is happening; only after a delay do we recognize what it is and assign it meaning. Similarly, if we decide to do something and our attention is diverted before action begins, we may retain only the sense that we intended to act, while the aim or even the movement itself is forgotten. A vague impulse remains, but its direction and goal are lost. Logically, the concept of a class follows the concept of the individuals composing it. Psychologically, however, class attributes are often known before individual attributes. Logically, one cannot grasp the notion of animal without first knowing vertebrates, fishes, mollusks, worms, and so on. Psychologically, one may have a clear idea of what an animal is without ever forming a clear notion of these subdivisions.

Knowledge of Other Selves

We describe mechanical phenomena and movements using terms borrowed from human actions, because human actions were noticed, named, and understood earlier. The same holds for mental life. We speak of semi-conscious and unconscious processes in terms drawn from conscious experience, and thus we are prone to mistake them for fully conscious processes. A psychologist who attempts to describe the dim, half-conscious intentions, feelings, and thoughts of introspectively undeveloped individuals is compelled to use language that properly applies to clearer processes in his own mind. He therefore describes others as if they were more conscious than they really are.

In this way, the psychologist unconsciously attributes to others the clarity of intention and thought he himself possesses. Just as an honest person believes others to be honest, or—if keen observation forces him to recognize their deceit—regards them as deliberate hypocrites, he finds it difficult to grasp the reality of self-deception, self-sophistication, and self-hypnosis—the capacity of human beings to mislead themselves into seeing people and things as their desires or interests require.

The pseudo-superior individual, who turns everything into a means for personal gain, cannot believe in the existence of genuinely superior men—those who love truth, knowledge, and art for their own sake, who take others' suffering to heart without calculation, and who argue only to reach truth, not to humiliate or exalt themselves. Such people appear to him either as incompetent pretenders or as eccentrics.

In our effort to understand the minds of other people, of animals, or even the nature of so-called inanimate things, we cannot avoid starting from our own inner life—just as we cannot reach a destination without first setting out from where we stand. To understand others, we must move in imagination either upward and forward, toward our aspirations and ideals, or backward and downward, toward our memories and earlier, more primitive conditions. Knowledge "from within," in the absolute or intuitive sense claimed by Bergson, is neither possible nor meaningful. Knowledge presupposes interaction between knower and known. Bergson alone appears to possess this secret, yet he refrains from revealing it; it suffices that he assures us of his possession of it.

The real danger in judging others by ourselves does not lie in beginning from our own experience, but in our laziness in remaining there. We fail to shift our standpoint, to compare perspectives, and to integrate partial views. We either identify others with ourselves, as children and philistines do, or we force them into the mold of our wishes, as exploiters do with the poor.

The productive individual, relying on his own abilities, initially assumes that others are like himself and treats them accordingly. Experience and objective thinking soon teach him otherwise. He learns to revise his assumptions, to cooperate with those of similar spirit, and to avoid parasites. The parasitical, predatory individual, indifferent to genuine knowledge and intent on living from the labor of others, persists in the belief that the poor are merely what he wishes them to be—tools, automatons, beings fit only for obedience. Those who resist and assert individuality he condemns as abnormal and seeks to destroy. He overlooks the fact that if independence-loving proletarians are abnormal because they are few, then his own class and its paid defenders—official psychologists and psychiatrists—are equally abnormal, being a minority as well.

The honest, creative thinker, by contrast, perceives in the oppressed masses not brute tools, but crippled souls—dimly aspiring human beings hypnotized into passivity by fear and exploitation. Those who profit from their labor deny them higher needs and even human feeling, because such denial best serves predatory and anti-social ends.

The same principles apply to our conception of the animal mind. The vegetarian, the kind-hearted, and the non-voracious individual is inclined to look upon animals with relatively unprejudiced eyes. Such a person readily perceives that animals, too, are stirred by passions—by fear and affection, hatred and love, joy and sorrow—and that they are capable of responding to gentle, fair, and loving treatment.

The fondness children show for animals arises not only because children—like our remote ancestors, whose life history each child briefly recapitulates—stand psychically closer to the animal world, but also because early humanity was predominantly vegetarian and therefore had no motive for denying a soul to its animal cousins. Denial of inner life appears wherever exploitation begins: just as exploiters deny humanity to the poor, and powerful nations deny it to exploited workers, so the flesh-eater finds it convenient to deny feeling and consciousness to animals in order to live without remorse upon their suffering.

Moreover, the child, like the primitive human being, tends to overestimate the mental life of animals by analogy with their often superior physical abilities. Conversely, the child finds it difficult to imagine a superior intellect housed in a small or physically unimpressive human body. The egoistic, voracious, flesh-eating individual, on the other hand, prefers to see in animals nothing but automatons, stored-up food or energy—much as carnivorous animals themselves, when driven by hunger, may look upon humans and herbivores.

To understand others, we must at some stage of our own development have been similar to them. For this reason, the most effective detectives and policemen are often recruited from among former criminals or those with a criminal predisposition. The most efficient servants are frequently found among aborted or would-be aristocrats. If the socialist is often better able than the innately gentle anarchist or communist to understand the mentality of a capitalist, it is because the socialist has passed, during his immature years, through a parasitical stage before reaching the humanitarian plane—at least in theory.

The capitalist who never evolves morally beyond the jungle stage remains incapable of understanding the socialist mind. Thus, writers such as Gustave Le Bon, despite scientific ability, fail when they attempt to analyze the soul of the socialist or the revolutionary. Whenever they appear to speak sensibly, they merely repeat ideas borrowed from socialist sources; whenever they speak in their own voice, they project onto socialists their own hidden traits—envy, fear of superiority, restless discontent, and hostility.

The intelligent person can understand the fool, and the sane person can partially understand the insane, because their own thinking passes through phases of vagueness, incoherence, impulsiveness, and subjectivity—but does not remain there. Thought is not allowed to pass into speech or action until experience has been consulted, sifted, clarified, and worked into coherent concepts or guiding principles.

The Organs of Knowledge

Just as in social life every complex task requires cooperation and division of labor among helpers, workers, supervisors, and initiators, so in individual activity every successful action requires cooperation among reflexes, instincts, habits, imitation, and individual initiative or reflection. There is no purely mechanical or purely manual labor. Even the simplest helper must employ attention, discrimination, and judgment; only the scope of reasoning differs. Hence, it is misleading to speak of "hand-workers" and "head-workers." It is more accurate to speak of simpler and more complex forms of work.

The same holds true of mental activity. Every mental process that aims at truth or objectivity requires the cooperation of senses, memory, intuition, spontaneous imagination, reflection, analysis, and synthesis. Sensation, perception, memory, imagination, and conception differ not by mutual exclusion, but by the number and complexity of objects involved. When a mental process is called perception rather than imagination or conception, it is not because the latter are absent, but because they remain in the background and play a subordinate role.

Up to a certain point, thinking and doing, feeling and expression, proceed together. Beyond that point they must separate and cooperate successively. The same applies within mental life itself. In simple matters, perception, memory, imagination, and conception operate simultaneously or in rapid alternation; in complex problems, they must act separately and in sequence. Passive perception, if allowed to dominate permanently, excludes active observation. Reproductive imagination must eventually separate from creative imagination if development is to continue.

Verbal and pictorial memory is inseparable from conceptual and assimilative memory in simple matters; but in complex affairs, the more attention we give to words, forms, details, and differences, the less clearly we grasp ideas, substance, unifying principles, and wholes. Since mental faculties cooperate either simultaneously or successively, and since each draws energy from the preceding one, no single faculty can be tested in isolation. Clear memory presupposes clear perception; clear perception presupposes understanding and attention; and attention itself depends on interest—that is, on spontaneous engagement rather than external compulsion.

Perception rests upon sensation; memory rests upon percepts; imagination rests upon memories; and conception rests upon imagination. Each higher faculty, like the upper stories of a building, rises upon those beneath it and offers a wider—though vaguer and more easily misleading—view of the world, of life, and of their possibilities. Thus we may remember things we can no longer directly perceive or feel; we may imagine things we no longer remember or have never perceived, things not yet perceptible, or even things that do not exist; and we may conceive things that lie entirely beyond the reach of both imagination and perception.

Had Kant kept this familiar psychological fact steadily in mind—had he not, like so many idealistic and nebulous philosophers, reached for clouds and empty abstractions while allowing the firm ground of experience to slip beneath his feet—he would not have entangled himself in what he called the four antinomies: those seemingly irreconcilable oppositions between finiteness and infinity, freedom and causation, contingency and necessity. Nor would he have felt compelled to offer a merely verbal reconciliation by dividing reality into noumenal and phenomenal realms. He would have seen that the infinite divisibility of matter, which imagination finds plausible because it pictures the invisible ultimate elements of matter by analogy with visible wholes, is exposed as absurd by reason. For infinite divisibility implies the existence of infinitely small particles—

particles of zero dimension—which is to say, particles that do not exist. For the sober, matter-of-fact thinker—who understands that all truth is necessarily relative, though not therefore arbitrary or unstable—there is no contradiction between necessity and freedom, between causality and contingency. A single event may be contingent with respect to one set of conditions and yet necessary with respect to another. More precisely, apparent contradictions arise only when opposite concepts are applied to the same thing in the same respect. A thing cannot be both greater and smaller than another thing, or both influenced and uninfluenced by it. But when applied from different points of reference, such concepts are neither contradictory nor harmonious—they are simply relational. To speak of the world as a whole as either necessary or contingent is, in fact, meaningless.

Our imagination cannot truly grasp the infinity or eternity of the world, but our conception can acknowledge them. Imagination often fails to show us that what is true of wholes need not be true of parts, and vice versa; reason, however, helps us to realize that although wholes are changeable and perishable, their ultimate elements must be eternal, indestructible, indivisible, uncaused, and uncreated. If everything had to be explained solely as the product of something entirely different, we would be trapped in an endless regress of causes, and the very notion of uncaused, spontaneous existence would lose all meaning.

All knowledge is relative or comparative; yet this does not mean that all knowledge is equally valid or unreliable. Only knowledge grounded in a stable point of reference, or in a practically constant unit of comparison, can be dependable, useful, communicable, and objective. If the temperature of our own bodies fluctuated wildly, as in a fever, our thermal nerves could never give us reliable information about changes in external temperature. Likewise, if our spontaneous inner activity oscillated violently without proportion to external stimuli, or were so explosive that the slightest impression transformed it entirely—as happens at times in highly emotional individuals—we could never attain adequate, objective, and differentiated knowledge of other people or of the surrounding world.

To gain such knowledge, our inner activity must possess a certain steadiness; its fluctuations must remain within limits, and the changes produced in it by external influences must be proportional to those influences. The irritable or explosive individual, who expects the world to conform to his wishes and needs and therefore never attempts to meet men and circumstances halfway, is inevitably condemned to illusion, disappointment, shock, and unhappiness.

All knowledge is knowledge of relations, of actions and interactions. There are no isolated, unrelated, inert things. Even latency and potentiality do not signify absolute rest or suspended motion; they indicate only imperceptible activity at molecular, atomic, or sub-atomic levels. The relativity of knowledge does not mean that truth can turn into falsehood simply because time passes or viewpoints change. It means only that knowing presupposes an observer situated at a particular point in space and time. If the observer's mood changes because of internal disturbances, or if his standpoint shifts, he has no right to conclude that the external object itself has changed.

Nor does the relativity of knowledge imply that knowledge is necessarily uncertain, fragmentary, or misleading. It means simply that we can know men, things, and ourselves only in relation to other men and things, only as acting upon and being acted upon. What appears as a complete individual from one perspective may appear as a mere part of a larger whole from another. Whenever many individuals act simultaneously, concertedly, and in the same direction upon another group, they effectively constitute a single whole.

From an extraterrestrial or abstractly philosophical standpoint, the conflicts among human beings may disappear from view, and humanity may appear as a single organism striving toward a common end and acting upon the external world in a unified way. Yet these conflicts, though invisible from such lofty perspectives, remain harsh and undeniable realities for human beings themselves, who live and suffer within them.

To expect knowledge and truth to exist independently of time, space, the human mind, and its points of view is to expect things to be motionless, unchangeable, inactive, homogeneous—in short, unreal. There is no such thing as absolute rest, absolute inaction, or absolute simplicity. Knowledge itself is a process, an activity of the mind, an interaction between the human subject and the external world. To say that things would still exist even if all human and sentient beings were to perish, and therefore cease to experience them, is simply to say that things would still act upon other things—that relations would persist. Existence is thus broader than being experienced: a thing does not cease to exist when it ceases to be experienced by human beings, but it would cease to exist if the rest of the world itself were annihilated.

Truth is nothing more than a collective or class name for all actual and possible sensations, feelings, perceptions, conceptions, viewpoints, and relations between them, as experienced by human beings and animals. If, instead of disputing in abstract terms whether absolute truth exists—that is, truth entirely independent of the human mind and of all relations—we were to descend to the concrete level of experience and ask a simple question, such as what color an object has in complete darkness or when it is not being looked at, we would quickly recognize the absurdity of the search for absolute truth.

Quantitatively, truth is more comprehensive than both knowledge and existence, for it includes actuality and potentiality, past, present, and future, and thus transcends immediate experience. Knowledge, by contrast, is coextensive with experience. Qualitatively, however, truth is poorer than knowledge, for it does not admit of degrees. Knowledge may be certain, believed, doubted, conjectural, or hypothetical; truth, as commonly conceived, allows no such gradations.

To claim that truth cannot transcend experience, or that the human mind cannot know anything a priori, is just as unreasonable as to claim that the mind can only react to the external world but cannot act upon it. Such claims deny the spontaneity and self-activity of the mind itself; they deny foresight and reduce knowledge to a mere record of the past, severing the vital link between past and future. Yet it does not follow, from the fact that human knowledge can transcend experience, that it can grow in any soil other than experience. All knowledge is empirical in origin—it draws its nourishment from experience—and at the same time transcendental in function, for it does not remain confined to past and present experience but surpasses them, anticipates the future, and helps to create new experience.

Potentiality

To clarify and define any concept, we must distinguish it from its superordinate, coordinate, and subordinate concepts; describe its scope and content; and trace its psychological genesis, which may coincide with its historical origin. Potentiality may be subsumed under the categories of existence or energy, depending on whether we consider it statically or dynamically. Potential existence is never detached from some form of actual existence: the tree exists potentially in the seed; forgotten ideas exist potentially in memory; before becoming conscious and dynamic, ideas exist in a structural, physiological, and unconscious form; combinations exist potentially within their elements. The concept of potentiality is invoked to explain hereditary transmission, the recall of forgotten experiences, the continuity of personal identity during sleep, and the restoration of disturbed equilibrium. Physiological energy contains psychical energy potentially; actions are contained potentially in abilities, thoughts, and feelings; a body occupying a higher position exists potentially in a lower one previously occupied. Ethical ideals exist actually in moral geniuses but only potentially in the morally average individual. Potential molar energy corresponds to actual molecular energy; when heat is added to a body, it first manifests itself in expansion—an effect perceptible to us—and later in changes of molecular structure that may be imperceptible.

To broaden the usual distinction between actual and potential energy, potential energy may be defined as energy of condition, and actual energy as energy of action. All impeded movement or restrained activity represents special cases of potential energy. Some have claimed that, for beings capable of freely moving through time as we do through space, the distinction between actual and potential existence would disappear. Yet this speculation collapses upon examination: if time were a form of space, sequence would become coexistence, and the very notion of temporal order would lose its meaning.

Related concepts to potentiality include latency, possibility, and immanence. Potential existence depends primarily on the inner, hidden qualities of the evolving entity, whereas possible existence depends more on external circumstances. Latency does not necessarily imply development, while immanence excludes efficient causation by external conditions. Potential energy accounts for energy not yet perceptible to our senses; latent energy explains energy that has ceased to manifest itself outwardly and is absorbed in internal work.

The concept of potentiality arises from the impossibility of conceiving creation out of nothing and from our need to think of causation as an unbroken chain. Viewed prospectively, potentiality explains evolution; viewed retrospectively, it clarifies causality and continuity; viewed aspectively, it accounts for what is imperceptible. In its naïve form, potentiality is conceived as being identical in nature with its later actuality, differing only in size or degree, while external conditions are thought to act merely as triggers. The more mature conception recognizes that the potential is itself a form of the actual, and that the realized outcome results from the interaction between the potential and external conditions—though the contribution of the potential is greater than that of the conditions.

In this way, human knowledge reveals itself not as a passive mirror of reality, but as a living process—rooted in experience, guided by reason, and constantly reaching beyond what is given toward what is still becoming.

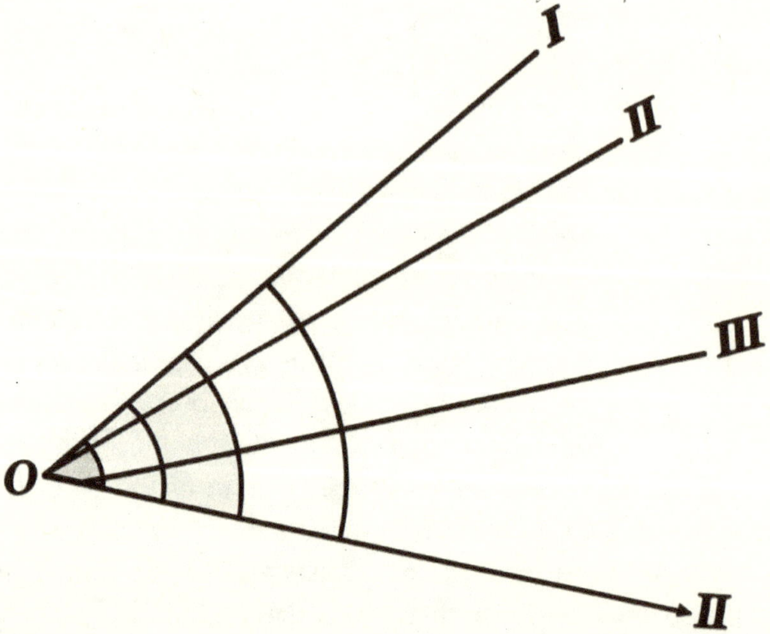

Just as the magnitude of an angle does not depend on the length of its sides, so the potential differences between individuals—between one person and another, between the genius and the philistine, between man and woman—are given congenitally. They do not change with age, nor with the outward growth of achievement. What changes with time is not the inner angle, but the distance between the sides. In the same way, actual individual differences—in quality, scope, and quantity of achievement—expand with age and development.

If all children appear alike, it is not because they truly are so, but because we are unable to discern, in their small present differences, the vast potential differences that determine their future paths. We lack the prophetic vision to see the future in the present, the great outcome in the modest beginning. We judge men not by their capacities and tendencies, but by their visible and momentary results; not by their reflected convictions, but by their memorized and professed opinions; not by what they genuinely think, feel, and do, but by what they imitate and pretend to think and feel.

Truth and Error

Theories, opposites, and ultimate categories of thought that appear irreconcilable from a fixed standpoint often reveal themselves, upon closer scrutiny, as mere abstractions—relative, interchangeable, mutually definable, and complementary—once the critical mind shifts its point of view. What, from a lower standpoint, is taken for reality, continuity, permanence, individuality, unrelatedness, quality, fact, absolute truth, beauty, or importance, may, from a higher conceptual standpoint, appear as appearance, discontinuity, instability, element, relatedness, quantity, relation, relative truth, ugliness, or insignificance—or may even vanish altogether.

Confusion, illusion, and error arise when knowledge gained from one standpoint is transferred uncritically to another and taken for what is seen there. The mind's eye, like the bodily eye, must first adapt itself to a new horizon. It must shake off disturbing after-images—after-thoughts and after-feelings—before it can see clearly again.

What holds for philosophy may be irrelevant for science, art, or practical life. What is real for the conceptual thinker, whose standpoint is existence in time, may be an empty word for the nominalist, whose standpoint is spatial existence. Not everything we know about mathematical space, time, number, or class can be applied indiscriminately to their physiological or psychological counterparts, or to individual beings. The real and the experienced are partly causes and partly effects of the imaginary.

Truth depends on three inseparable factors: the observer, the object observed or imagined together with its setting, and the point of view. If truth appears identical for different observers, it is so only to the extent that they themselves are alike.

By this, I do not mean—like pragmatists, instrumentalists, and other philosophically inconsistent minds—that there are many kinds of truth, that truth is merely subjective or identical with utility, or that what is true for one person or one science must be false for another. I mean only this: the whole truth is not accessible to every person, at every time, under all circumstances, from a single standpoint. What is seen from one perspective is only a part of the whole truth. It may be invisible, irrelevant, or obscured from another perspective, yet it is not antagonistic to it—only complementary.

Memory and imagination enable us to synthesize these partial truths into a more comprehensive unity. They complete immediate experience, fill its gaps, compensate for the limits of perception, and spare us the need for exhausting and minute observation.

To ask for absolute truth—truth independent of observers, of relations, of settings; truth about things-in-themselves—is to indulge in a verbal illusion. It is equivalent to asking how a thing looks when no one looks at it, or how a thing would appear if nothing else existed in the universe. Such questions are empty plays of words, as meaningless as asking how a man feels when he is dead, or where the light goes when a candle is extinguished.

We constantly mistake the imaginary for the real, the dream for waking life, the abstract for the concrete, words and symbols for thoughts and things. We confuse the inanimate with the animate, the unfamiliar with the personal, the new and individual with the old and habitual, the conventional with the natural. This happens because imagination and dreams are distorted copies of reality; because abstractions never exist apart from the concrete; because words originally tied to bodily and visible things are later used for mental and abstract processes;

and because habitual, inherited ways of thinking demand less effort than new, individual, acquired ones.

The ultimate sources of error and illusion are mental inertia, fatigue, laziness, habit, distraction, and preoccupation. Under their influence, knowledge, feelings, and attitudes formed under old, familiar, narrow, and personal conditions are transferred wholesale to new, unfamiliar, broader, and more objective situations—or the reverse—without adjustment. In this uncritical transfer lies the persistent root of human misunderstanding.

In mature life it becomes difficult to separate the direct and immediate data of the senses from the corrections and additions supplied by inference, memory, imagination, and subconscious reasoning. Yet, in moments of distraction—when the mind is absorbed in associative or centrally arising processes—we may occasionally glimpse what peripherally incoming sensations are in themselves, and thereby what they must have been in early childhood. In such moments of absorption we sometimes catch ourselves believing that two objects belonging to different planes lie in the same plane. This reveals that pure visual perception does not originally contain distance or solidity; these qualities are later products of subconscious inference.

Abnormality does not consist so much in the mere experiencing of illusions as in the despotic persistence of error; not so much in reacting to illusions as in reacting inadequately; above all, in indulging simultaneously in mutually exclusive illusions. Just as ignorance and erroneous opinions—unlike stupidity and prejudice—are curable, so the illusions of the sane differ from the delusions of the insane in that the former are corrigible, whereas the latter are incapable of rectification.

Since reason—apperception, memory, imagination, conception, understanding—is only an extension and refinement of the senses, it is improper to make either reason alone or the senses alone the exclusive judge of reality and truth. The true criterion of truth lies rather in the agreement between sense and reason. Only in matters that are indirectly accessible to the senses—such as electrical phenomena, past or probable events, distant occurrences, the microcosm and the macrocosm, and the minds of others—must reason alone serve as the criterion. Conversely, in simple, habitual, normal, and constantly recurring experiences, the senses by themselves may safely be entrusted with the judgment of reality.

The lowest senses—the so-called chemical senses of smell and taste—give us limited information about a small number of substances, and only when parts of these substances are absorbed by the corresponding nerves. The mechanical senses—muscular, thermal, tactile—provide richer information about innumerable bodies, but only when these bodies act directly upon our nerves. The sense of hearing operates at a distance through a relatively coarse medium, such as air, liquids, or solids. The sense of sight reaches much farther still, through the most subtle medium, long conceived as ether.

Memory and imagination enable us to complete present experience and to anticipate future experience. Conception allows us to survey, with minimal time and effort, vast fields of experience without attending to every particular instance. It also enables us to know things that act indirectly or imperceptibly upon our senses.

Under normal conditions, all our senses reveal reality with varying degrees of adequacy. The older senses—tactile and muscular—disclose the more general, stable, and primary properties of things, such as pressure and weight. The later-acquired senses—sight and hearing—reveal more particular, changeable, and secondary qualities, such as color and sound. Under unusual conditions, the senses interpret new experiences in terms of old ones, thereby giving rise to illusions. These illusions are corrected either through sensory adaptation or through reasoning in the light of past experience.

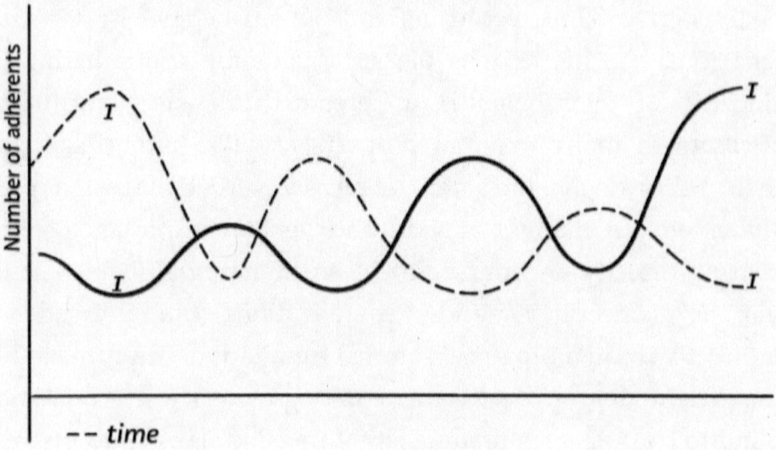

1. Frequency curve of materialism, monism, realism, mechanism, sciences, etc. 2. Frequency curve of spiritualism, dualism, idealism, vitalism, religion, etc.

Truth of Opposite Theories

It is exceedingly difficult to decide, by statistical methods, which of two opposing philosophical views is in the ascendancy and therefore the true one. To determine this, we would need to know the number of genuine adherents of both positions—I and II—at successive historical periods, in order to construct their respective frequency curves and to infer from them the general tendencies of decline or growth, assuming that truth ultimately prevails.

A simpler and more convincing proof of the truth of II, however, lies in the fact that, at a more advanced stage, many professed adherents of I act in practice as though they were adherents of II. True convictions, as we know, reveal themselves more clearly in action than in verbal professions. There can be no real compromise between the two positions. Compromise is possible only in words, not in deeds.

This is not to deny that a person may profess I while acting according to II, owing to inner disharmony, timidity, suggestion, or hypocrisy. Thus, preachers and devout believers often cling tenaciously to life and its pleasures, thereby contradicting the sincerity of their belief in a hereafter. Likewise, spiritualists attribute so many material properties to the human soul that their belief degenerates into a merely verbal idol or a party shibboleth. In matters of vital and general importance—those bearing directly and immediately on human well-being—truth, that is, conceptions and generalizations built directly or indirectly upon a broad sensational foundation, can be tested by the general degree of agreement among men. Those who remain blind to truth in such matters either perish or lapse into insanity. But in matters that bear only indirectly, remotely, or imperceptibly upon human well-being—in scientific and philosophical questions—agreement among many is no reliable test of truth. One person may be right while thousands are wrong. Truth steadily gains adherents; error may also gain temporary dominance, but it cannot maintain it indefinitely. Thus, the fact that scientist after scientist and philosopher after philosopher attributes to ether all the general properties of matter except weight does not prove that ether is weightless. They forget that if ether appears imponderable, it is because we live immersed in an ocean of ether, from which we cannot escape, and within which all worlds float. Air, too, would appear imponderable if we had no means of creating a vacuum and weighing a vessel before and after removing the air. The same holds for water: its weight cannot be measured by scales immersed within it. Weight, being a special case of attraction between two bodies at a distance, cannot be measured directly when that distance is zero, even though the attraction may then be maximal. Cohesion and attraction are known through the force required for separation. If we could separate ether from other substances and from the earth, we might determine whether it has weight. In the same way, individuals often fail to realize the depth of their attachment to one another until external circumstances threaten to separate them.

Belief, Doubt, and the Law of Conservation

Originally, we are inclined to believe, to accept as real, objective, permanent, constant, and absolutely true whatever we experience or are told. Doubt—and with it the distinction between reality and appearance, objective and subjective, absolute and relative, permanent and changeable—is imposed upon us by increasing knowledge and by contradictions arising from later experiences concerning the same objects. A new theory that shatters belief in an older doctrine also undermines confidence in its own implications. The microscope, for instance, destroys not only our belief in the homogeneity of the cell, but also our belief in homogeneity and continuity in general. Just as a slanderer undermines trust not only in others but also in himself, so the destruction of one belief weakens belief as such. Our ultimate concepts lose their former absoluteness; yet belief in their relative validity becomes, in a certain sense, absolute—it transcends the experiences from which it arises. We believe in persistence and constancy as long as we do not encounter change. When belief in the persistence of known things collapses, we transfer it to hidden forces, noumena, unknown substrata; from there it is transferred again to a hypothetical primitive substance or energy of which all actual substances and forces are taken to be manifestations.

The law of the conservation of matter and energy is not so much a law of nature as an approximation to it—a mental instrument for understanding the world. It is as much a product of our mind, of our aspirations and desires, as of objective experience. It may be regarded as a corollary of our instinct for psychical and bodily self-preservation. When permanence in the external world comes into conflict with permanence of the self, we sacrifice the former to preserve the latter, admit miracles, or modify our conception of immortality—shifting from the immortality of the bodily and conscious individual to that of the dynamical, psychical, or cosmic principle. It might equally be argued that our instinct of self-preservation is itself a mental aspect of the cosmic law of persistence. The mature thinker comes to recognize that body and personal mind are perishable. The only way in which our thoughts, feelings, and tendencies achieve permanence is by becoming impersonal, common property, detached from individual embodiment.

Truth, Beauty, Utility, and Morality

Corresponding to the three constituents of every state of mind—cognition, affection, and volition—there are three qualities in objects: reality (or unreality), beauty (or ugliness), and utility (or harmfulness).

Reality refers to the essence, the permanent and hidden qualities of things, and reveals itself in sensation, perception, and conception. Beauty refers to form and appearance, to those changeable qualities that intensify our vital rhythm or gratify general life-needs, and it manifests itself in feelings of pleasure. Utility refers to the capacity of things to satisfy particular needs, to fill deficiencies in our psycho-physical organism.

By extension, beauty is attributed not only to objects that directly gratify vital needs, but also to those that symbolize or foreshadow favorable, life-enhancing conditions. Hence, beauty is rightly ascribed to moral intentions. Entirely unjustified, however, is the mystical identification of beauty in general with the ethical. Not only external objects arouse states of mind; states of mind themselves may become objects of thought, memory, or imagination. In such cases, a thought is true if it rests on a sensational foundation; beautiful if it harmonizes with a broader system of mental states; useful if it leads to greater stability and a richer or more intense life; and moral if it serves the community, group, or species to which we belong. Just as idea, feeling, and will are irreducible to one another, so reality, beauty, and utility are irreducible qualities. They may cooperate, but they may also diverge. A concept may be true without being beautiful or useful. Illusions are often beautiful and temporarily useful. Truth is not always useful—indeed, it may be harmful to certain social classes—but it is never harmful, and often beneficial, to humanity as a whole. For this reason, the capitalistic philosopher—the pragmatist or sophist—and the church-bound philosopher—the scholastic—are inclined to reject truths that do not serve the interests of the exploiting class. They conceal this selfish criterion beneath the respectable language of social value. Truth, however, is always allied with intellectual usefulness for the genuine truth-lover, for the person to whom knowledge has become not merely a means, but a vital need and an aim of life.

Truth from the Capitalistic Point of View

If the disclosure of truth depends upon the mental constitution of the observer and upon the standpoint from which he views life, it follows inevitably that the capitalist's conception of existence, of human relations, of society, and of the world must differ profoundly from that of the proletarian. From this it further follows that the class struggle—the concealed war carried on between the capitalistic, parasitic, predatory class and the laboring masses in the economic, industrial, and political sphere—is only one outward expression of a far deeper psychical, and often physical, difference between these two types of men. This struggle, properly so called, cannot be successfully understood or overcome if it is studied in isolation from its other manifestations on the intellectual plane—religion, ethics, philosophy, art, and literature.

The productive, social class can no more afford to accept the false and narrow doctrines devised by capitalism, or its distortions of broader and truer doctrines, than it can afford to submit to the intolerable economic conditions imposed upon it. Capitalism and socialism are not merely opposing economic systems; they are antithetical and mutually exclusive philosophies of life, ethics, art, and modes of struggle for existence. The predatory human being, who merely consumes, destroys, and obstructs production, must of necessity hold a conception of himself and of his fellow-men entirely different from that of the productive, creative, and peaceful individual. Indeed, the conceptions of the exploiter—voiced by his spokesman, the pseudo-superior man—are the direct opposite of those of the producer, as expressed by the genuine superior man.

What appears true and good from the capitalist's narrow, selfish, predatory, local, and momentary standpoint is inevitably false and harmful when judged from the socialist's broader, humanitarian, constructive, cosmopolitan, and enduring point of view. Many genuine superior men have been prevented from attaining a clear understanding—still more from developing an original conception—of a consistently socialistic philosophy, ethics, or world-view, owing to their dependence on capitalistic publishers, patrons, and employers, and to the influence of capitalistically biased friends, audiences, readers, and educational institutions. Moreover, the fact that among intellectual proletarians interest naturally spreads more widely in history, economics, and literature than in philosophy, psychology, and ethics—fields that demand greater leisure and preparation—explains why the former disciplines have been, and are being, rewritten from a socialist standpoint, while the philosophically inclined proletarian minority must vainly attempt to quench its intellectual thirst at the inaccessible, exhausted, and contaminated well of academic philosophy.

Capitalists and their dependents regard their less fortunate fellow-men as living tools or as dull beasts of burden that must be driven to work by compulsion, fear, intimidation, or deception—by flattery and cajolery. Judging others by himself, by his own inability and unwillingness to produce, the active parasite behaves as though the earth were too small for all, as though nature were a stepmother, as though poverty resulted from overpopulation rather than the reverse, and as though the means of existence were scarce and non-multipliable, to be seized as quickly as possible. He is therefore a natural admirer of war, both in its primitive military form and in its modern, disguised, competitive form, since he reaps the benefits without risking his own life.

Even an eminent sociologist such as Lester Ward, while admitting the widespread reign of deception, greed, and parasitism, finds nothing blameworthy in them. On the contrary, he defends them as inevitable and as morally unconscious as a destructive lava stream. He fails to perceive the horror and devastation of war, because, as a member and defender of the predatory class, he sees only its immediate and selfish advantages for his own group.

The predatory individual lacks the sense—and therefore the understanding—of universal kinship and cooperation, of the unifying and strengthening power of love, of the ultimate superiority of truth over falsehood, and of the far-reaching constructive possibilities of cosmopolitanism. He who denies the existence of class struggle and class differences when their ugliness is exposed by socialists is often the first to propagate beliefs in "blue blood," aristocracy of birth, divine rulership, and the alleged rewards of innate superiority. He accentuates his separation from the toilers while professing their equality.

To him, life is a clever game of deception and outwitting others. The world is a stage for the display of theatrical talent, not a field for the fulfillment of duties or a mission. His notion of altruism is a verbal simulation; at best, it signifies moderation in predatory behavior, never its abandonment. His relation to the deity he imagines is conceived as a business transaction—an exchange of what costs him little for something of greater imagined value. Intelligence, in his eyes, is the ability to deceive others, to gain their favor cheaply, and to secure their support.

He cannot conceive of intellectual or humanitarian pursuits as ends in themselves, but only as means to fame, wealth, and bodily comfort. Anyone who finds genuine happiness in disinterested intellectual or humanitarian activity appears to him as a fool or a crank. Religious and moral practices are, in his view, good only insofar as others adhere to them. Language itself is, for him, an instrument for concealing his intentions and weaknesses while compelling others to reveal theirs. Virtue is something to be simulated and demanded of others; vice is something to be practiced secretly while discouraging it publicly.

Truth, for him, consists of opinions that it is advantageous to hold—or at least to profess. Social service, leadership, and cooperation mean noise, command, and self-important bustle, while the real work is left to others. In capitalistic language, a "good man" is one who can be easily deceived, silenced, or bribed.

Capitalistic art and literature are romantic, sensational, morbid, effeminating, superficial, and playful rather than realistic, penetrating, serious, instructive, or elevating. Capitalistic science is biased, exclusive, formal, often a mere display of wit or an instrument of exploitation rather than an earnest search for truth and socially beneficial invention. Capitalistic ethics is double-faced and sophistical, designed to obscure the true nature of social organization and to conceal or idealize the predatory and demoralizing role of the so-called upper classes.

Capitalistic philosophy is a distortion and caricature of the genuine philosophy taught by the great thinkers of humanity. It is lifeless, barren, verbose, nebulous, and enslaved to words; estranged from daily life and from the marketplace, to which Socrates, Jesus, and other genuine philosophers brought philosophy. Its function is to lull its adherents into dreams of self-conceit and imaginary superiority over the masses.

Capitalistic charity, reform, government, and administration of justice are largely a farce—mere pretexts for cruelty, exploitation, or corruption, or cheap devices for pacifying and deceiving the oppressed. Corresponding to their moral duplicity, capitalists and their clerical and intellectual allies employ a double vocabulary: exaggerated praise for themselves, euphemisms for their own crimes, and denigrating terms for their victims. Their language is vague, ambiguous, evasive, and distorted, diverted from its natural purpose of conveying ideas.

When the capitalist extols liberty, laissez-faire, competition, private enterprise, and initiative, he does not mean what individualist thinkers have meant by these terms—the free and fair exchange of services among capable and willing individuals. He means simply the unrestricted right of deceitful and parasitic persons to prey upon producers. In the same way, when a sexual parasite speaks of a single moral standard for both sexes, he does not mean equal demands of purity, but equal license for exploitation.

Thus, truth, as conceived from the capitalistic point of view, is inseparable from power, advantage, and predation; whereas from the social and humane standpoint, truth is bound to cooperation, justice, and the progressive liberation of human life.

The reasoning displayed by the exploiter whenever his privileged position is threatened will be an inexhaustible source of amusement for future generations. It would already be amusing to us, were it not that we ourselves must pay so dearly—often with our health, freedom, and even our lives—for the follies and fallacies of this logic. To the exploiter it appears perfectly natural that he should be entitled to an easy, comfortable, and happy existence. What he cannot comprehend is why modern workers, instead of gazing up at him with envy, do not console themselves for their poverty by looking down upon paupers, or by looking back to ancient times when even kings never dreamed of comforts that many workingmen now possess.

That he himself has been accustomed to luxury from early childhood seems to him a sufficient justification for preserving his privileges. That the poor, too, could become just as quickly accustomed to comfort and security, and might desire them with equal right, never strikes him as a valid claim.

He perceives no wrong and feels no remorse when he wastes his life in idleness and the pursuit of pleasure while his fellow-men toil, ruin their health, and cripple their minds in exchange for bare subsistence. It never occurs to him that there is anything criminal in enjoying the fruits of other men's labor while deliberately avoiding work himself. Yet he is indignant when some destitute man dares to enjoy even a fragment of what he has not produced.

If the idler despises labor and looks down upon the man on whose work he lives, this seems to him natural and free of ingratitude. But if a starving man shows no reverence for usurped property, this is branded an atrocious crime demanding the harshest punishment. Well-fed, idle parasites—protected by laws they themselves have made or had made for them—prey with impunity upon the entire nation, yet see nothing absurd in sitting in judgment over a hollow-cheeked wretch who, driven by hunger, has stolen from a single individual. They regard it as their unquestionable right to judge the poor, whom they daily rob of health, liberty, dignity, and life itself. But when the oppressed attempt to judge the decrees and actions of their masters, this is denounced as insolence and "contempt of court."

The capitalist, or his prostituted spokesman—the pseudo-superior man—declares that workers have only themselves to blame for their misery: their lack of ability, ambition, thrift, or foresight. He never pauses to consider that even if every worker were equally gifted, they could not all become supervisors or overseers. The parasitic aristocrat prides himself on his ancestors' supposed merits or services, yet it never occurs to him that a descendant who lacks such qualities ought to renounce unearned privileges and feel ashamed of occupying them. He boasts of tracing his pedigree farther back than that of the toilers, as though their ignorance of ancestral names implied that they sprang spontaneously from the soil, or that they do not share the same remote human or prehuman ancestry.

The American parasite, or the parasitically inclined simpleton, feels superior to immigrants merely because he was born on American soil, as if the land or air possessed some mystical power to ennoble the mind, or as if its chemical composition differed from that of other countries. He does not carry his reasoning far enough to recognize the Indigenous inhabitant as the "true" aristocrat, since that inhabitant inhaled more of this supposedly ennobling air than he ever did. It seems self-evident to him that men who do not speak his language must be inferior and uncivilized, while the fact that his ignorance of their language and customs could just as well be taken as proof of his own inferiority never troubles his self-satisfied logic.

When the exploiter robs the poor under the shelter of laws and contracts in whose making the poor had no voice and no real choice, his conscience remains untroubled. Yet he would leap in outrage if it were pointed out that he is morally worse than a highway robber who bluntly says, "Your purse or your life." His behavior is, in fact, equivalent to that of a hypothetical robber who, before plundering his victims at gunpoint, politely requests them to sign a written agreement consenting to be relieved of their valuables.

To the parasite it is axiomatic that he is entitled to extract the greatest possible reward for the least possible service—even for mere noise or sham work—and that he is fully justified in squeezing from his employees the last drop of energy, provided they have "agreed" to it. Whether this agreement was extorted under the pressure of starvation, homelessness, or the threat of the workhouse does not concern him. The intellectual prostitute—the academic lecturer, preacher, journalist, official scientist—finds it perfectly natural to be handsomely paid for platitudes, recycled ideas, or stolen and diluted thoughts. Yet he mocks with merciless contempt the poor genius who seeks to live by his originality and dares to believe that sincere poetry, heartfelt stories, altruistic social ideas, or fertile thoughts deserve public support.

When moral geniuses arise who take to heart the suffering and degradation of the masses and attempt to awaken them, prostituted academic psychologists and psychiatrists hasten to the defense of their patrons. With arrogant certainty they brand these men as abnormal, morbid, eccentric, or maladjusted—simply because they differ from the majority, remain indifferent to material success, or disregard social approval. They forget to apply the same logic to themselves and to their masters, who also form a minority, and one that acts against the interests of the majority—thus having an even stronger claim to be labeled pathological.

The exploiter never doubts that he is a useful member of society and that without his orders the world's work would come to a standstill. Yet he cannot provide any clear standard by which his usefulness could be measured, either quantitatively or qualitatively. When the socialist proposes that the value of commodities and the remuneration of services should be determined primarily by the amount of useful labor expended or social labor saved, the exploiter immediately denounces this standard as impractical, unjust, arbitrary, and incapable of accounting for individual differences or qualitative distinctions. That the labor standard, despite its difficulties, stands immeasurably higher than the arbitrary, fluctuating, and socially destructive commercial standard lies beyond his narrow field of vision.

That men who have never performed a stroke of socially useful labor should be entitled to bequeath vast fortunes—titles to the fruits of others' toil—does not strike the parasite as absurd or criminal. But that men who have worked and suffered all their lives should leave their children destitute and defenseless in a predatory world seems to him perfectly compatible with logic and morality. In his view, the only reprehensible theft is the taking of property without the owner's verbal consent. He cannot perceive that a far greater crime is the monopolization of common property—land, water power, forests, mines, public offices—through the consent of bribed officials who have no right to dispose of what is not theirs, or the enslavement of fellow-men by a consent extorted under the threat of starvation or imprisonment.

The problem of unemployment offers little difficulty to the capitalist logician. He solves it swiftly: unemployment is caused by the unfitness of the unemployed, and the remedy lies in training, vocational education, or the elimination of the unteachable. It never occurs to him that under a system of private monopoly the number of applicants must always exceed the number of available positions—even if all were equally capable. Still less does he realize that in an age of extreme specialization, division of labor, and machine production, talk of general "unfitness" is sheer nonsense.

Thus the logic of exploitation reveals itself not as ignorance alone, but as a deeply rooted psychological distortion—one that serves privilege by turning injustice into virtue, usurpation into right, and human suffering into a convenient abstraction.

Quantity and Quality

Quantity and quality are correlative terms: they are inseparable, and neither can be reduced to, nor fully expressed in terms of, the other.

Yet just as the fact that the terms father and son are correlatives does not prevent a father from being, in his own turn, the son of someone else, nor a son from later becoming a father, so the correlation of quantity and quality does not mean that what is quantity in one respect, or in relation to certain objects, cannot at the same time appear as quality when viewed from another angle or in relation to other objects.

Matter and energy (or motion) form such an inseparable pair of quantity and quality. Matter, however, presents itself in innumerable combinations which, from certain points of view, differ so widely that they are regarded as differences in kind, as qualitative differences of substance. Motion, in turn, is both quantity—magnitude, velocity, acceleration—and quality, in the form of direction. Different motions may combine in such ways as to give rise to energies that are qualitatively distinct. Time and space form another inseparable pair of quantity and quality.

Time clearly admits of quantitative subdivision, and it may be that space itself arises from qualitative syntheses.

Differences between varieties of the same species appear, from a lower, emotional, practical, and narrow standpoint, as qualitative differences, differences of kind. From a higher, more intellectual and theoretical point of view—when the varieties of one species are compared simultaneously with those of other species—the same differences appear as quantitative, while the distinction between species becomes qualitative. From a narrow outlook, the pursuits of superior men seem entirely different from those of philistines; from a broader, more philosophical or timeless standpoint, these pursuits differ only in quantity, in the remoteness and scope of the goals pursued.

In its advanced and complex human form, mind appears as an energy sui generis, apparently unrelated to mechanical energies and seemingly exempt from their laws, such as conservation or equivalent transformation. Yet future inquiry may succeed in tracing all energies back to a common origin from which they diverge. It is possible that studies such as those of Jacques Loeb on tropisms may help to illuminate the origin of mind.

Does the Actor Create?

The so-called genius of the actor consists chiefly in the power of auto-hypnosis: in the ability to evoke the consciousness of a particular personality, to identify with it, and to act accordingly. This imaginative power presupposes, as Nordau has pointed out, an undeveloped, unstable, or shifting personality in the actor himself—a mind with a movable center of gravity, a changeable nucleus of dominant interests.

Through the persistence of infantile imitation and through constant observation of emotional outbursts in himself and others, the actor acquires voluntary control over emotional expression, gesture, and posture. This control is often reinforced by autosuggestibility—the hysterical capacity to summon and combine emotions, and to identify oneself with dramatic or living characters.

The actor must therefore be placed among the lowest class of artists: the purely emotional, reproductive, formal, and juvenile type. He expresses through his own face, movements, and voice the same emotions and passions that the painter or sculptor expresses through external material. In the same way, the dancer arouses emotions through rhythmic bodily movement that music seeks to evoke through vibrations of air.

The actors of the future will not be recruited from hysterical or epileptoid individuals whose unsettled personalities allow them to impersonate many roles. They will be normal individuals. Economic independence will enable them to represent primarily characters of their own type—idealized or caricatured versions of themselves. Acting will then be a vocation rather than a profession. Modern commercial theaters, however, cannot afford such actors; they require individuals willing to live irregular, nomadic, and lax lives, and capable of playing many roles.

All pseudo-superior men—professional moralists, preachers, orators, politicians, leaders, rulers, organizers—belong to the same class as actors, or what might be called imitative geniuses. The difference between stage actors and those of the pulpit or platform lies mainly in this: the latter usually play only one role and can therefore maintain greater inner balance. Another difference is honesty. The stage actor does not wish to be mistaken for the character he portrays; the pseudo-superior man does. The priest or rabbi—especially the reformed rabbi—or the professional ethical culturist poses as a moral genius; the politician as a patriot or reformer; the professor or journalist as an original thinker; the head of a charitable institution as an altruist. The kinship between actors and pseudo-superior men is so close that in countries relatively free from rigid tradition, such as the United States, it is not uncommon to see actors become preachers or politicians, and preachers or politicians become actors.

Authorship

The thinker or genius becomes an author when his scattered and fragmentary thoughts find a central idea around which they crystallize, as crystals form around a nucleus. In the merely erudite author, only the central idea is original; the remainder is compilation, or at best an original method of exposition. Such authors proceed systematically and methodically; they can appreciate the far-reaching implications of original truths but lack the power to discover them. The author of genius, by contrast, reaches original conclusions with ease, often without being fully conscious of how or why.

In the poet, emotional commotion—inspiration—brings ideas and sentiments into contact, all converging toward a single emotional effect. The dominant emotion selects and attracts only those ideas or aspects of ideas that can be focused upon a common center. The originality of the poet lies less in the ideas themselves than in their arrangement and in the language that expresses them. Hence the absurdity of turning poetry into non-poetical prose.

There are two kinds of aphoristic writers. Some write in aphorisms because they are unable to think a problem through in all its aspects, or because they lack the learning needed to bridge the gaps between their flashes of insight and the fuller context supplied by others. Such writers often overestimate the value of their isolated aphorisms because the larger framework that would give them proportion is missing. Others write aphoristically because they dislike verbosity, repetition, and the dressing of simple truths in scholastic or rhetorical finery. They prefer to present the germ and gem of truth without adornment. If their aphorisms later prove to be fragments of an organically growing intellectual structure, they willingly shape these fragments into a harmonious whole, rather than leave them as raw material for other, broader-minded architects.

Original knowledge is drawn primarily from personal observation and experience—from the School of Life—under the catalytic influence of ideas acquired from other original minds. This explains why the works of geniuses contain relatively few quotations. The writings of merely talented men, composed largely of common truths restated with slight modifications, are heavily interspersed with quotations—often unacknowledged, especially when the original authors lack fame or the means to defend their intellectual property. While originality tends to coincide with minimal imitation, the absence of quotations does not necessarily prove originality; it may also reflect unconscious imitation, purely verbal novelty, or the expression of anonymous commonplaces.

The clear-headed thinker does not feel compelled to write until he has reached definite conclusions. He does not burden his readers with the wanderings, errors, and trivialities through which his thought has passed. The nebulous, inconsistent, or mystical thinker, by contrast, begins to write and teach before achieving inner clarity. He hopes that truth will reveal itself in the very act of expression, and therefore communicates everything that crosses his mind, leaving readers to separate the valuable from the trivial, the true from the false, according to their own inclination.

The less original a writer's central idea is, and the less clearly it is grasped by the author himself, the greater is his inclination to indulge in lengthy preliminaries, formal classifications, and methodical digressions. He talks around the subject without entering it, circling endlessly without reaching the core or moving in medias res. The poorer the intrinsic value of an author's opinions, the more carefully he postpones their presentation to the expectant reader, and the more eagerly he places them in "good company," that is, amid venerable and authoritative doctrines. He hopes that the unquestioned reverence accorded to these time-honored views will cast some reflected glow upon his own meager ideas.

The truly original mind acts otherwise. It speaks directly and moves straight toward the mark. It dispenses with superfluous introductions and avoids obscuring the central idea beneath ornate language, paradoxical turns, artificial complexity, or attention-distracting verbal embellishments. Nor does it conceal the main thought within an imposing display of erudition designed to impress or mystify. Even at the risk of being accused of dogmatism, the original writer hastens to present his general conclusions and supports them—where support is needed and possible—by a small number of typical, well-established, personally observed, and easily verifiable facts.

The writer who loves truth disinterestedly does not beat cautiously around the bush, nor does he dramatize his own importance. He goes straight to the point. He does not selfishly hoard insights that could never have been reached without the collective intellectual inheritance transmitted by earlier generations. Unlike the pseudo-superior man, he does not keep his readers in artificial suspense or inflame their curiosity merely to heighten the effect of his "revelations." Nor does he linger over his ideas to impress others with profundity or originality. He does not choose words for their pleasing sound, nor does he attach exaggerated importance to a rigid order of exposition.

The selfishness, vanity, idleness, dream-indulgence, formalism, appearance-hunting, superficiality, conventionalism, word-idolatry, and deceptiveness of the parasitical ruling class are faithfully mirrored in the literature, philosophy, and certain sciences—such as economics, sociology, theology, and history—produced by their hired artists, academics, historians, priests, and moralists. In contrast to the honest thinker, the capital-dependent and mercenary writer often strives deliberately not to be understood. His aim is not to convey ideas in clear, popular language, but to intimidate readers into admiration, and to weaken their confidence in their own judgment and intellectual capacity.

The pseudo-critical, unfair, or intellectually dishonest critic habitually ignores or minimizes the strong and convincing points of the doctrine he attacks—its original contributions, practicable consequences, and genuine merits. Instead, he fixes attention exclusively on weak points, nonessential defects, unoriginal elements, formal or linguistic shortcomings, and speculative difficulties of little real significance. His occasional praise is insincere and restricted to trivial details, serving merely to lend credibility to his destructive intent. He condemns social, ethical, or religious movements in the name of humanity, civilization, patriotism, liberty, or general welfare, while in reality he is defending the interests of his own class, party, or clique. He denounces theories and works of art in the name of truth, logic, and objectivity, while his real motive is personal ambition, jealousy, or hostility toward their authors.

The honest and genuinely original thinker, by contrast, defines his terms clearly and distinguishes unambiguously between his own views and those he criticizes. He does so not because he imagines that words possess fixed and immutable meanings, or that sharp boundaries exist between what is one's own and what belongs to others, but because he is sincerely devoted to truth and justice. He is prepared to defend or to abandon his position in accordance with the impartial judgment of human reason. He willingly assumes not only the credit but also the responsibility and possible blame attached to his claims.

The dishonest, sophistical, fame-seeking, and self-advertising writer behaves differently. He avoids clear definitions and carefully refrains from precisely formulating his own theses. By doing so, he gains freedom to encroach upon the intellectual territory of others while jealously guarding what he proclaims as his own. This strategy allows him to appropriate ideas that rightly belong to others or that have already become common intellectual property, and to reap credit without exposing himself to responsibility, refutation, or accountability.

A single example may illustrate this method of intellectual dishonesty. In his defense of free will, Henri Bergson declares the concept to be indefinable. By this sophistical move, he leaves himself free to appropriate facts that properly belong to determinist explanations. At the same time, he conveniently obscures the boundary between time and space, shifting back and forth between these conceptual domains whenever his position becomes vulnerable. In this way, he seeks refuge in one domain when his weaknesses or artifices are exposed in the other.

End of the Chapter

Chapter-5.
Affective Life:
Solitude, Sympathy, and Inner Companionship

This chapter examines the emotional life of superior individuals—why they often walk in solitude yet remain inwardly rich, how they experience deeper pain and deeper joy, and how true companionship is found not in crowds but in shared devotion to truth, beauty, and moral purpose.

Solitude

Although endowed with abundant vital energy, the superior individual suffers deeply—and this suffering leaves lasting marks—when he is compelled to abandon the well-worn paths of common life, to part with the cherished illusions of the average person, and, after casting them aside, to set out alone on an untried road and venture upon untrodden ground.

Yet in another and deeper sense, the superior person is never truly alone. He carries within himself a vast inner world of thoughts and feelings; in imagination he shelters both the ages that have passed and those yet to come, and he communes with the noblest minds of humanity through the ideas they have left behind.

Common mortals, by contrast, fear solitude and dread the company of their own inner world, which is for them an empty desert; hence their restless flight into external amusements and distractions.

What renders the superior person so solitary in this world is the fact that those who love him do not understand him, and those who understand him are strangers to him. His loneliness is therefore twofold: he is separated from the common masses who live on planes far below his own, and he is also separated from other superior individuals who, though moving in the same sphere, rarely follow the same paths.

If thinking were the rule and the goal of life, and not merely an exception or a means for the majority, thinkers would not be condemned to solitude; they would not be rari nantes in gurgite vasto. Thoughtless activity—such as games and idle diversions—and unrestrained imagination—such as wit and playful poetry—are far more sociable than logical thought. To become sociable, the thinker must imitate others and approve uncritically what they do or say; he must, to some extent, deny his higher self. The novelist and the psychologist who draw their creative impulses from society are more sociable than thinkers who derive theirs from the inanimate world; and even they are most sociable during the phases of conception and communication, not during the period of incubation and creation, which demands solitude and undisturbed concentration. The novelist concerned with particular human events is more sociable than the psychologist who seeks the laws governing human thought, feeling, and conduct. The ethical psychologist, the moral critic who strives to uncover the hidden motives of human action and the psychological roots of social evils, must maintain an even greater distance from his fellow men than the non-ethical psychologist. Excessive intimacy and community of interests blur moral vision and obscure the general drift of ethical problems. The unfortunate individual endowed with both intellectual and moral genius feels isolated alike among the intelligent few and the philistine masses: he values the masses for their frankness, simplicity, and unspoiled moral core, yet their ignorance and dullness distress him; he appreciates the educated for their grasp of higher aims, yet his warm and sincere heart chills in their selfish and hypocritical atmosphere.

The moral genius, above all, strives to keep aloof from character-destroying and ideal-stifling organizations, parties, and cliques whose sole aim is the pursuit of power, authority, and privilege. He prefers to observe them from a safe distance, to infer their intentions from occasional signs, and to compel them to honor their promises by fearlessly exposing their evasions and deceptions. He educates the people—either directly as an agitator or indirectly through his writings and readers—to keep control over their supposed representatives and to demand tangible results.

Most unbearable to the intellectual and moral genius is the company of aristocratic and would-be aristocratic philistines, who combine egotism, vanity, cold-heartedness, greed, envy, and malice with stupidity, emptiness, dullness, and slavish devotion to form and convention. His penetrating insight into human nature—his ability to read indifference or hostility behind friendly words, to discern what is left unsaid behind what is spoken, and to distinguish courtesy from genuine friendship—renders him, much to his regret, less expansive, less effusive, and less eager for society. This reserve, however, differs fundamentally from the affected stiffness, conceit, and selfish aloofness of sham aristocrats and pseudo-superior individuals.

The superior person is often unjustly accused of misanthropy because he avoids philistines. By the same logic, the great mass of average people could be called misanthropic, since they do not feel at ease in the company of thinking individuals. The idealist passes through life in loneliness, making few, if any, genuine friends, because he demands from others the same depth, purity, and sincerity of affection that he himself offers. He willingly sacrifices quantity for the sake of quality.

If love of truth and reflective thought were the norm rather than the exception, the genius would not be solitary; he would feel at home among his fellow men. The pseudo-superior individual, by contrast, is only seemingly sociable. Outside of exploitation or demagogic aims, he keeps his distance from the masses and regards them with contempt. Even when he approaches them, he does so with condescension and simulated kindness, carefully reminding them of the favor he bestows and of his supposed superiority, maintaining psychological distance despite temporary physical closeness. He takes pleasure in his slight intellectual advantage over the ignorant and therefore strives to keep them in a state of stagnation. Horace speaks for such pseudo-superior men when he declares, "Odi profanum vulgus et arceo." Had he spoken for genuine superior individuals, he might have said, "Ama profanum vulgus sed arceo." When the genuine superior individual keeps his distance from the masses, it is not from hatred or contempt, nor from pleasure in being different. On the contrary, he is pained by the fact that the masses remain under the influence of pseudo-superior leaders and have not yet reached the level required to understand him and to follow his clear and direct path toward brighter and happier regions. Instead, they allow themselves to be led by profit- or fame-seeking guides who prefer tortuous and obscure routes in order to prolong their own importance and render their leadership indispensable.

Similarly, when the intellectual genius avoids close association with women, it is not due to misogyny or morbid hostility toward the female sex. Rather, it pains him that so few women are yet prepared for genuine intellectual companionship.

He simply cannot breathe in a philistine, materialistic, and prosaic atmosphere. When an exceptional genius appears to delight in female society, it is usually due to sensuality, vanity, or both, rather than to higher motives. Far from being a woman-hater, the man of genius regrets that the female sex has produced only scattered and isolated figures of intellectual stature, such as Aspasia, Cornelia, Mary Wollstonecraft, Rahel Varnhagen, George Eliot, Olive Schreiner, Ellen Key, Ida M. Tarbell, Charlotte Perkins Gilman, Clara Zetkin, Elizabeth Gurley Flynn, Emma Goldman, and Mother Jones.

Communicativeness and unrestrained talkativeness, when not confined to rigid conventions, are signs of sincerity and genuine sociability, and are often found among proletarian philistines. When the genuine superior individual, though honest and eager to share knowledge, appears less communicative, it is not because—like the hypocritical pseudo-superior person—he lacks sociability, has little to say, wishes to conceal his individuality, or speaks only for advantage. It is because he pursues serious aims and detests empty talk on conventional subjects merely to pass the time. He prefers meaningful discussion, yet recognizes that his words will often fall on unresponsive ground. Moreover, unlike the philistine whose audience is limited to neighbors and acquaintances, he also has access to the written word. He therefore consoles himself for the indifference of those around him with the hope of reaching, through his works, sympathetic readers scattered across the world and among future generations.

Pain, Pleasure, and Emotion

That individuals of higher intellectual and moral development feel moral pain more acutely than the average person does not render their lives bitter. On the contrary, they are equally more sensitive to moral, aesthetic, and intellectual pleasures. Their inner emotional resources are abundant, enabling them to find consolation and meaningful compensation for loss. Even if the only pleasures available to them were those of creation, these alone would more than repay every renunciation demanded of them.

The intellectual joys of creation are naturally accompanied by certain physical or nervous strains. Yet in a well-balanced superior mind, these leave no lasting harm—just as the pains of childbirth do not destroy a physically healthy woman and are more than compensated by the deep and enduring intellectual joys of motherhood.

Wisdom does not lie in suppressing or destroying emotion; it lies in governing emotion through reason. In the superior individual, emotions and affections are intellectualized. They are less violent and less explosive than those of the average person, but they are more enduring, more stable, and more conscious of both their origin and their purpose. Such a person is not irritable or impulsive; rather, he is sensitive and reflective. His convictions are not fanatical or intolerant, but steady and broad-minded. What he loses in sudden intensity, he gains in duration. Emotional energy, instead of erupting destructively, is channeled and distributed usefully across the whole of life. Rather than being exhausted in a single moment or opportunity, it nourishes all experiences over time.

He avoids extreme emotional exaltation, in which the soul loses equilibrium despite concentrating all its energy on a single aim, and where even a slight shock can cause a collapse into the opposite extreme. He equally avoids depressive emotions. Both forms—exalting and depressing—are intoxicating and equally destructive to mental and physical balance.

The principal current of his aesthetic pleasure changes its course. It moves away from the narrow field of raw sensation and perception toward the realm of ideas and concepts, from the concrete to the abstract, from the familiar to the unknown. When certain geniuses appear to lack aesthetic taste, this may simply mean that their aesthetic sensibility has been wholly transferred to the sphere of broad ideas and abstract truth. The child or the primitive mind delights in sounds and colors; the youth, the ordinary individual, and the sentimental temperament delight in perceptible forms—paintings, statues, and visible beauty. The thinker, however, finds beauty in a theorem, a scientific law, a social structure, or a philosophical synthesis. Higher aesthetic pleasure does not necessarily abolish lower forms; it may coexist with them.

The genuine intellectual individual possesses a direct, disinterested, and self-sacrificing love for knowledge. He loves truth for its own sake, as an end in itself. The pseudo-intellectual, by contrast, loves knowledge only indirectly and conditionally—only insofar as it serves personal advantage, ambition, or vanity. When conflict arises, he is prepared to distort or abandon truth altogether. The intellectual philistine remains openly indifferent, or even hostile, to abstract and impersonal knowledge. At best, intellectual activity becomes mere play or purposeless occupation for the pseudo-superior individual and the philistine alike.

The same distinction appears in the moral realm. The genuine altruist loves others sincerely and without calculation, often forgetting himself in the process. The pseudo-altruist loves conditionally—only when such love aligns with personal interest. The moral philistine is frankly indifferent to the happiness or suffering of others. To love truth or humanity disinterestedly does not necessarily mean to love them more than oneself, although such devotion is sometimes found. It simply means to love them for their own sake, as ends in themselves, not as means—present or future—to personal gain. The balanced intellectual individual is frequently mistaken for an egoist and judged less altruistic than he truly is. This misunderstanding arises because greater altruism is expected of him than of ordinary people; because he pays little attention to minor material comforts, whether of others or himself, particularly when absorbed in intellectual work; because his altruism is more passive than demonstrative, more general than personal. He loves humanity broadly rather than confining his concern to a small circle of familiar individuals. His interests and commitments are divided among many pursuits, and he expresses affection less visibly than he feels it. He lacks the time and patience for trivial expressions of sentiment, conventional gestures, and socially expected displays on conventional occasions.

A barking dog is far less dangerous than one that bites silently from behind. The same holds true among human beings. The ordinary individual or impulsive philistine, who quickly becomes irritated and openly vents anger, is socially less harmful than the pseudo-superior person who conceals resentment and patiently prepares revenge, striking unseen and undetected. The most socially valuable individuals are the genuinely superior ones, who neither indulge in irritation nor harbor thoughts of revenge, but simply despise wrongdoing openly and withdraw from those who practice it.

The same motive that drives a dog—before and after stealing a bone—to hide or assume a threatening posture is rooted in guilt and fear: fear of being discovered before the act, and fear of losing the stolen object afterward. This same psychology explains the predatory philistine's narrow range of base emotions and his distorted behavior. At its core lie unsociability, inaccessibility, excessive caution, secrecy, selective alliances, fear of intimacy, suspicion of strangers, and hostility toward harmless individuals. From this source arise his tendency to interpret social movements as mere envy, his inclination toward veiled coercion and bluffing, his distrustful nature, his incapacity for genuine friendship or love, his assumed air of superiority, his aversion to fearless and critically minded individuals, his morbid sensitivity to criticism, his vindictive resentment, and his eagerness to disguise parasitic aims under the language of social service.

Courage of the Will

The courage of the ignorant and of the mentally unbalanced arises from an exaggerated belief in their own power combined with an underestimation—or complete ignorance—of external resistance. Such courage therefore collapses rapidly and is soon followed by deep discouragement. The courage of the vain or pseudo man of action takes a different form: it seeks to impose the will upon others through unscrupulous and dishonest means, in order to convince both others and himself of its supposed strength.

The true man of action, however, prefers obedience freely chosen over obedience imposed. His strength of will is sustained by the conviction that the direction of his effort serves socially useful ends. He knows his own firmness and perseverance too well to need the humiliation or subjugation of others in order to feel powerful. At the same time, he is fully aware of the magnitude of external resistance—physical as well as social—and therefore avoids premature enthusiasm or self-congratulatory triumph. These distinctions apply equally to intellectual courage and emotional courage. The naïve individual expresses opinions or feelings boldly because he is unaware of opposing views or assumes that others think and feel as he does. The self-conceited individual forces his convictions and emotions upon others, not because of their intrinsic truth or worth, but because of self-adoration and vanity. The intellectual courage of the genuine thinker flows from the compelling force of objective truth, while the emotional courage of the poet arises from the universal, impersonal, and enduring value of his emotions. The courage of the naïve ignores obstacles and therefore does not avoid them. If by chance such a person encounters no resistance, contradiction, or visible disapproval, his courage persists. The courage of the pseudo-superior individual is maintained by evasion—by ignoring, circumventing, intimidating, bribing, or removing obstacles and opponents. In contrast, the courage of the genuinely superior individual lies in facing resistance openly and striving to overcome it honestly and definitively, whether that resistance appears as selfishness, indifference, inertia, wounded vanity, ignorance, or superstitions deeply intertwined with cherished human sentiments.

Wisdom and Aspiration

The truly superior individual remains inwardly consistent amid life's changes and reversals; he does not lose balance at the heights of glory or fame. Only the artistically superior temperament tends toward capriciousness and irritability. In such cases, the lower reflex centers are weakly connected to the higher sensory and intellectual centers, allowing emotional and impulsive reactions to dominate reflective judgment. This dissociation may be permanent and structural, or temporary and dynamic, arising when intense mental absorption prevents higher centers from regulating peripheral emotional currents, or when exhaustion weakens their controlling influence.

Human happiness often conflicts with nature's rhythm. We seek permanence, continuity, and essence, while nature offers change, transience, periodicity, and form. These fluctuations disturb only shallow spirits. The superior individual is liberated from vanity through an understanding of the constant transformations of human destiny.

Wisdom represents ambition in its mature form. The ambitious individual desires not so much to be superior as to appear superior and to be honored. The wise individual seeks to be—to become inwardly complete—and finds satisfaction within the tribunal of his own conscience. The desire to please others is not a direct motive for him; the judges whose approval he values are not transient and unthinking crowds, but the clear-minded and impartial thinkers of all times and places.

As intelligence develops, the objects of aspiration evolve. Higher stages of development seek values that are more enduring and less vulnerable to circumstance. Apathy gives way to vanity, vanity to ambition, and ambition to wisdom. Emptiness of mind yields to curiosity, curiosity to a thirst for knowledge. Respect for outward form is replaced by respect for inner substance. Sentimentalism gives way to reflection. Cowardly or foolish reluctance to judge others gives rise to gossip and malicious criticism of individuals, which in turn is transcended by social criticism, ethical psychology, and the disinterested study of human types and their influence on the progress and welfare of humanity.

Morality and Social Achievement

Average morality is largely a product of circumstances. Superior morality, by contrast, is a force that transforms circumstances and creates new social conditions. The individual of superior morality remains moral despite adverse surroundings, while the moral philistine acts morally only when circumstances permit or demand it. Unlike jurisprudence and conventional ethics, which limit themselves to overt actions and immediate consequences, ideal ethics also considers thoughts, intentions, emotions, and tendencies, as well as remote and indirect effects, insofar as the individual is conscious of them. Moral philistinism, as reflected in jurisprudence, judges conduct from narrow, immediate, personal, and class-bound perspectives. It focuses on declared intentions and conspicuous but secondary effects. It exhausts itself in prosecuting individual offenders and relies almost exclusively on laws, courts, police, and armies—institutions that can only respond to crimes after they occur and that address only the visible symptoms of social disorder. Their guidance rests on precedents that can be distorted, traditions devoid of substance, and arbitrary rulings by a few self-appointed authorities.

Moral genius, expressed through social ethics, adopts a fundamentally different standpoint. It evaluates human activity according to vital and general interests—social welfare and collective happiness—guided by reason, logic, and common sense. It refuses to remain satisfied with legal punishment or superficial reform. Instead, it investigates the deepest causes of crime and suffering and seeks the means of preventing them. It concerns itself with human types rather than isolated individuals, with lifelong patterns rather than momentary acts. It identifies social, anti-social, and parasitic forms of life, examines the effects of occupations and activities on society, and therefore calls for radical reform of economic, political, and social institutions.

This ethical vision does not demand the mere reformation or elimination of criminals; it demands the abolition of a predatory system that produces and multiplies them. It rejects the belief that order can be maintained by appointing a small, corruptible group to police vast populations. Instead, it holds that justice and social order are best secured by entrusting responsibility to all—by cultivating goodwill in every heart and self-control in every mind. To moral genius, the immense and intricate legal machinery of the present appears as a pitiable makeshift, destined to remain ineffective so long as it leaves untouched the predatory economic foundations of society—so long as profit-seeking and privilege-hunting dominate, so long as production serves profit rather than general use, and so long as the fundamental human right to meaningful employment is denied.

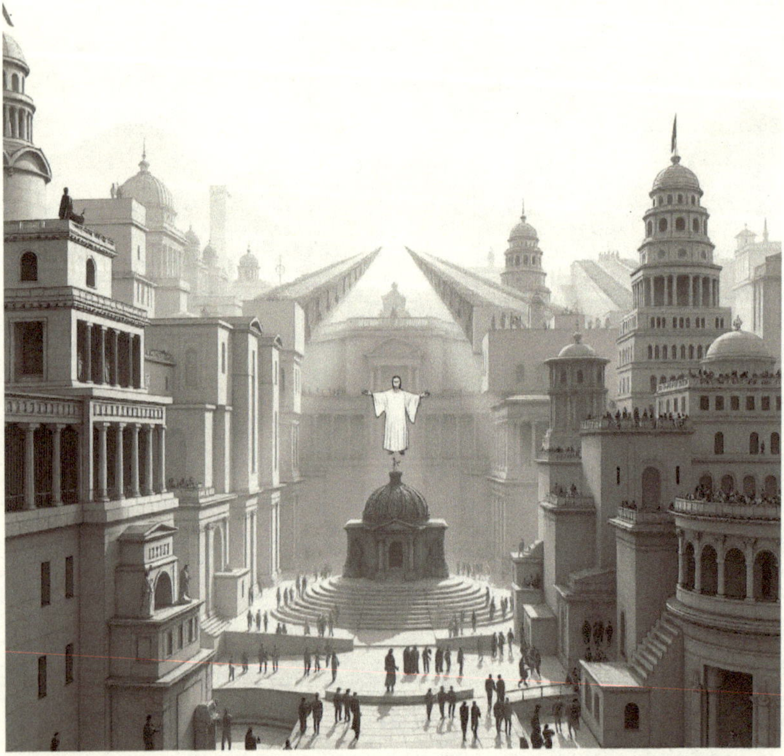

When legislation finally embodies these principles, it will be prepared to free itself from the tangled growth of confusion and pseudo-complexity that now overwhelms it. Law will return to its original, rational simplicity: a small body of clear, common-sense rules, resistant to distortion by legal sophistry and immune to the verbal ingenuity that thrives on ambiguity.

Superior morality is not the exclusive possession of intellectually superior individuals. It appears at both ends of the human spectrum: among simple, honest working people and among those of great intellectual power. It is rare at the extremes in the weak-minded and in narrowly one-sided geniuses, and rarer still in the middle range of intelligence—among the merely "clever" and the conventionally talented.

Just as water flows from higher to lower ground, so wealth flows from the higher moral level of working people and truly superior individuals toward the all-absorbing lower moral level of the "smart set" and the talented. In the animal world, the strong survive; within human society, however, it is often the self-seeking, the hypocritical, the cunning, and those protected by them who succeed. Only in an ideal society founded on solidarity would selection favor the morally superior.

What the moral genius recognizes as duty is regarded by ordinary humanity as sacrifice or exceptional merit; what he considers a crime does not yet fall within the limits of accepted ethics. The average moral individual calls himself good if he performs his duty, allows the world to continue in its accustomed course, and refrains from directly contributing to the increase of human misery. The moral genius, by contrast, condemns our indirect and unintentional participation in injustice. He even condemns passivity itself—our role as indifferent spectators to the tragedies enacted daily on the world's stage. He finds it criminal to enjoy life's pleasures while remaining conscious of the countless heart-rending sufferings endured by our fellow human beings, fellow citizens, and collaborators in the creation of our comfort.

He denounces as immoral those rulers, scientists, poets, professors, journalists, and professional talkers who offer nothing but words of compassion to the dispossessed working class where decisive action and courageous struggle are required to secure truly human conditions of life. Truth in social matters does not come from those comfortably placed within society and benefiting from it. It comes from outsiders—from moral geniuses who lead a quasi-extra-social existence, excluded from the banquet of so-called sociable people. Only these moral outsiders are able to survey society as a whole, across space and time, and recognize that it has lost its way. Only these disinherited moral figures can hold before humanity the image of its own distorted and criminal face, foresee the fatal consequences of its false direction, and raise the warning cry in time.

Morality varies inversely with the intensity of our striving for success and external possessions. It is therefore easier for a person devoted to self-perfection to attain the highest moral levels than for one driven by ambition. The saying "Tout comprendre, c'est tout pardonner" applies only to superior individuals. For others, it would be more accurate to say, "Tout oublier, c'est tout pardonner."

What self-control and self-consciousness are for the superior individual, public opinion is for the average person. The former is governed from within, the latter from without. Public opinion serves as a substitute for, and a precursor to, self-control—just as politeness is a substitute for, or a forerunner of, love and genuine sympathy. Under the modern competitive system, with its vast, complex, unsolidary, and uncontrollable communities, authority, leadership, and success do not fall to harmoniously developed, wise, altruistic, and well-balanced individuals. Instead, they go to the degenerate and one-sided, to men of a single pursuit, to usurpers, the greedy, the unscrupulous, hypocritical cowards, self-appointed authorities, the morbidly vain, the bluffers, and the hunters of appearances. These are the ones who succeed, rule, and control the means of existence, thereby imposing their standards of living and behavior upon the masses.

If superior individuals often appear timid, awkward, indecisive, inactive, unsociable, unfit for money-making occupations, or incapable of gaining popularity, it is because they lack the deceptive skill and disguised aggressiveness—

euphemistically labeled diplomacy, histrionic ability, self-confidence, or entrepreneurial spirit—of commercial philistines and pseudo-superior figures. They prefer to deal with people and matters thoroughly, conscientiously, and wholeheartedly. They reject reliance on ready-made phrases, conventional gestures, and stereotyped manners that superficially suit every occasion. They refuse to respond verbally and emotionally in a shallow, mechanical way to the appeals of others, nor can they accept such empty responses in return for their own genuine expressions of feeling.

They are less inclined than seekers of notoriety to engage in public activity where there is no real prospect of achieving something meaningful, let alone fulfilling promises made to the people. Their seriousness of mind and devotion to higher intellectual and unselfish aims prevent them from feeling at ease among frivolous, materialistic, pleasure-seeking individuals, whether socially or professionally. They are too straightforward, frank, open-hearted, and fair-minded to adopt the crooked, hypocritical, cowardly, and predatory practices of the business world—by which is meant a world in which everything, including commodities, religion, knowledge, and philanthropy, is reduced to commerce—or of so-called Society.

Nor do they easily succeed with the honest but intellectually blind masses of working philistines, who mistake the demagogue's flattery for friendship, his promises for goodwill, his theatrical heroism for real courage, and, in general, his pretenses for reality.

Happiness and the Desire for Approval

Many-sided development protects the self-respect of the superior individual from degenerating into megalomania, for it reveals to him how small his actual abilities are in comparison with those he does not possess or possesses only to a limited degree. The happiness of the ordinary person consists in living in harmony with instinct, habit, and tradition, in following well-trodden paths. The happiness of the superior individual lies in opening new ground for future generations. The philistine experiences inner emptiness when he departs from routine; the superior individual suffocates within the narrow confines of philistine monotony. The philistine becomes frightened and disoriented when invited by a superior mind to abandon conventional grooves and venture into the vast, unexplored fields of possibility—fields rich with promise for those who dare to explore them.

The balanced superior individual, whose critical sense is not distorted by vanity or impulsiveness, knows both his strengths and his limitations. He is therefore difficult to humiliate and less vulnerable to insult or lack of recognition. The ordinary person, lacking an inner standard by which to judge himself, depends entirely on external approval—praise, admiration, or envy—to assess his worth. For this reason, he suffers deeply when he is criticized, ridiculed, ignored, or rejected by others.

In pseudo-superior individuals and in philistines, self-knowledge and self-esteem are determined chiefly from without. Such persons respect themselves only in proportion to the respect shown them by others. The slightest sign of disrespect is enough to shatter their self-confidence; their self-love becomes deeply wounded and persistently irritated. They therefore avoid situations where esteem is uncertain and actively seek occasions for flattery. Directly or indirectly, they pay for compliments and crave praise they have not earned. Because they are poorly convinced of possessing genuine worth or superior ability, they require constant reassurance from others. They strive to please at any cost, particularly those who pose as critics or admirers, in order to receive approval in return. Unable to command respect through authentic personality or real knowledge, the pseudo-superior individual seeks substitutes—titles, ranks, diplomas, symbols of distinction, social position, affectations of mystery, secrecy, and eccentric manners—in the hope of achieving outward recognition.

The exaggerated self-esteem of the megalomaniac is subjective: it tolerates no greater personalities, does not grow gradually through achievement, and is ostentatious, egotistical, and often cruel. The self-esteem of the genuinely superior individual is objective. It rests on knowledge of one's own merits and on comparison with the achievements of others. It grows in proportion to the increasing manifestations of originality and creative power. It is inclusive, restrained, and modest rather than demonstrative.

In the balanced superior individual, intellectual courage and self-confidence increase with deeper knowledge of oneself, of others, and of the world; with growing originality; with accurate foresight; and with hypotheses repeatedly confirmed by experience. In parallel, there is a steady decline in suggestibility—that blind, uncritical obedience to what others say, command, or do.

The genuine intellectual creator, unlike many professional scholars and institutional authorities, is less sensitive to criticism and takes no offense at refutation. He loves truth for its own sake, and he knows that his merits are numerous and solid enough to be recognized sooner or later. He therefore has no need to pursue unearned recognition and finds no difficulty in accepting limitations imposed by nature.

Similarly, the moral creator, unlike professional moralists and reformers who turn ethics into an occupation, can afford to have intentions, feelings, and actions criticized. He knows that genuine moral worth cannot be destroyed by attack, and he has no material interests bound up with moral preaching. Unlike the philistine, who lives entirely absorbed in the present and sees little beyond the narrow circle in which he moves, the creator lives in and for the future. He anticipates the distant and the potential, which are more real to him than the immediate and the actual. The philistine magnifies momentary pleasures and momentary troubles alike, lacking a sense of proportion. He has never reached the imaginative heights from which the present, the recent past, and the near future—his entire world—appear in their true, fleeting insignificance. What seems to him colossal, fearful, and overwhelming shrinks into transience when viewed from these heights.

The creator is not crushed by poverty, obscurity, ridicule from contemporaries, or persecution by exploiters. Like the explorer or the missionary, who is compensated for the scorn of hostile surroundings by the esteem of a few companions and by the thought of distant gratitude, the pioneer of the future perceives, beyond present contempt, the admiration of generations yet unborn. He can already enjoy, in anticipation, the freer and happier life of those who will one day benefit from paths opened by such despised visionaries as himself.

His idea of immortality is not the philistine's naïve fantasy of bodily resurrection. It is intellectual immortality—the lasting influence of ideas, discoveries, and higher aims impressed upon future generations. The absence of domestic happiness does not empty his life of meaning, for he finds consolation in the vision of a future form of companionship, for which he seeks to prepare the ground: a partner economically independent, intellectually equal, and capable of true collaboration in life.

He is not surprised that superior individuals rarely find fulfillment in marriage within existing conditions. After long ages of social stagnation and isolation, the sexes have drifted so far apart that mutual understanding of higher aspirations has become rare. This fact does not lead him to despair of humanity. Living amid countless morally and intellectually stunted forms of life, he still finds solace in imagining a nobler, more generous, and broader-minded type of men and women who will flourish under cooperative conditions—conditions toward which the small, scattered, and often persecuted group of moral creators continues to strive.

End of the Chapter

Chapter-6.
Life Under Striving:
Between Mammon and Meaning

This chapter confronts the tension between a life devoted to gain and a life devoted to meaning. It explores why many struggle endlessly for Mammon while a few strive for inner truth, showing how thought, action, and ideals collide—and how authentic fulfillment arises only when striving serves higher purpose rather than mere survival.

In the Realm of Mammon

1. Ah, how life unfolds in the great city here:
Struggle without pause, relentless striving,
Self-interest, envy, and greed.
Human tides surge forward,
Hardly knowing where they go—
Storm-driven, untamable,
Now here, now there.
    Everything rushes,
Granting itself no rest.
"Soon—just a little longer,"
One keeps saying,
"We shall reach the goal,
Happiness will be attained."
Yet how endlessly many
Are so easily destroyed
In the confusion of life,

Where, without respite,
One struggles, struggles in vain
Against the heavy burden of desire.

2. Truth alone, and love:
If these were to remain
Our striving here on earth,
Then—and only then—
Could there be true happiness below,
Granted equally to all.

O. L. S.

Berlin, October 19, 1901

Theory and Practice.

The theoretical individual perceives successively what the practical individual apprehends at once. To profess a principle in theory does not imply the ability to realize it in practice. Practice is the resultant of many forces that rarely act in the same direction: theory, emotions, habits, instincts, and external influences. Theory is not simply another form of practice; it is most often its complement. The less idealism there is in action and conduct, the more idealism is professed in theory. What is lacking in lived practice is compensated for in proclaimed convictions and self-suggested doctrines. If theory were merely a translation or mental equivalent of action, we should expect the highest degree of idealism, altruism, moral progress, and tolerance among priests, preachers, moralists, religious devotees, orators, and leaders—and the least among materialists, atheists, and plain people. Experience shows, however, that the opposite is frequently the case.

In individuals whose inner life is unharmonious or disharmonious, the convictions they profess—often reinforced by self-suggestion and expressed in speech, manners, or outward appearance—form the complement of their actual practice, which in turn reflects the operation of their habits and instincts.

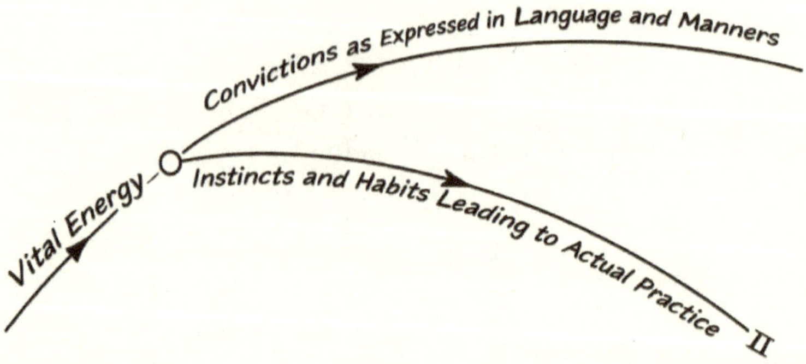

In symbolic form this relationship may be expressed as: (C + P = V; C < P; CoL + M + … ; P ∝ H + I).

In harmonious and morally balanced individuals, convictions, habits, and instincts converge and act together in conduct. This harmony may be represented as: (C + H + I = O; P ∝ V; C ≤ P).

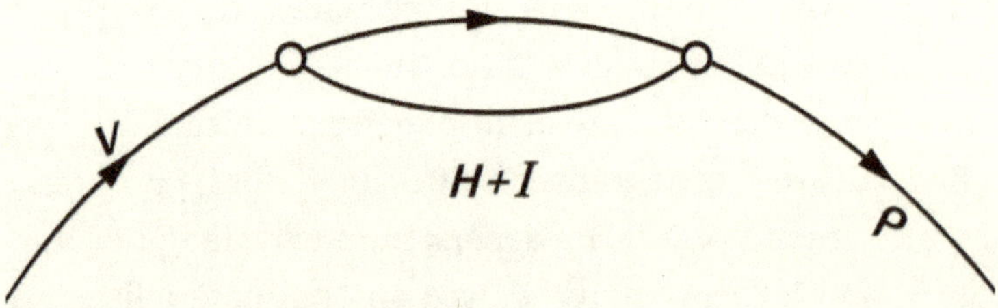

The majority of people live in direct contradiction between theory and practice. Their theories are impressed upon them from without—through suggestion, imitation, and the influence of superior minds—while the motives guiding their actions arise from within, through heredity, habit, and ingrained instinct. Only the genuinely superior individual lives, to any significant degree, in harmony between thought and action. All wise truths have long since been spoken, all wise maxims have already been preached, and they are found on everyone's lips—even on those of the foolish. Yet only the wise individual acts in accordance with them; only the ideal individual takes them seriously into the depths of his life.

So weak is the connection between thinking and acting among philistines, and especially among pseudo-superior individuals, that those who most loudly preach—whether in books, editorials, sermons, or speeches—honesty, idealism, poetry, chastity, and virtue, very rarely act honestly, ideally, poetically, or purely. On the contrary, as a rule, they live dishonestly, materialistically, and prosaically. And the reverse is also true: those who glorify dishonesty, theft, violence, crude realism, or sensuality seldom act accordingly; more often than not, they behave with outward correctness and restraint.

This observation is not meant to suggest that the moral sermons of dishonest hypocrites are entirely without value, nor that the glorification of cruelty, egoism, or vice by individuals who are mentally but not practically perverted is therefore harmless. The point is rather a simple and important one: for the welfare of human society, it is better to deal with individuals who are consistent—whether virtuous or vicious—who act as they think and preach, whose influence is visible, definite, and constant. The consistently vicious individual is less dangerous because he inspires little trust and is more easily recognized. The consistently virtuous individual is more useful, because he demands not merely verbal agreement but practical commitment to the principles he teaches.

Those who feel an urgent need for inner consistency and for the approval of others, and who therefore attempt to justify or defend actions that run counter to custom, law, or public opinion, are usually harmless and ineffective. They betray themselves through hesitation, regret, and excessive explanation, and often confine their originality or immorality to words alone. Far more dangerous are those who instinctively, quietly, and resolutely act in selfish and immoral ways, without any need for verbal defense or rationalization. Such individuals conceal the ugliness of their conduct—both from others and from their own distorted conscience—by loudly professing moral principles.

This disguised anti-social type publicly proclaims unconditional respect for abstract principles, blind faith in authority, confidence in the impartiality and goodwill of appointed guardians of law and order, belief in the automatic triumph of truth and justice, and trust in the power of well-worded laws and promises regardless of who formulates or enforces them. At the same time, in practice, these individuals show the least loyalty to their professed ethics. Secretly and instinctively, they violate moral and legal codes, flatter and bribe those in power, conspire, court influence, purchase favors, submit themselves servilely to authority, and tyrannize, exploit, blackmail, persecute, and undermine those who naïvely trust in the incorruptibility of institutions or the inviolability of laws and constitutions.

Our capitalist, predatory social system has no use for harmoniously developed, many-sided, and fully human individuals. Such individuals cannot easily be reduced to tools for monotonous, degrading labor, and their idealism, altruism, visions, and theories tend to assume clear and concrete forms that demand realization. In doing so, they threaten the interests of those engaged in exploitation. Far more welcome to the ruling classes are intellectually crippled or narrowly developed philistines who willingly serve as tools, as well as the inharmonious, muddle-headed, or hypocritical pseudo-superior individuals whose idealism is vague, lifeless, playful, and safely confined to words. Their theories are so detached from their actions and instincts, so harmless and ineffectual, that they pose no obstacle to predatory interests and may even serve them.

Thinking and Acting

Because the principal source of their happiness lies within themselves—in their creative power—it becomes clear why balanced superior individuals often appear less restless, less outwardly active, than those whose happiness depends on others, on recognition, success, wealth, or applause. The superior individual carries everything within himself (omnia secum portat). In reality, he strives no less than the ambitious person, and often far more; but the results he achieves are less visible, less immediate, and less easily measured by external standards.

The intellectually superior individual strives toward lofty ideas and ideals, yet he rarely fights directly for their realization among the masses. This task falls instead to emotionally richer individuals—agitators, leaders, reformers, and statesmen. The truth-loving, many-sided, contemplative thinker generally leaves the practical realization of ideals to emotionally charged, single-minded, enthusiastic, often naïve reformers, as well as to unscrupulous, self-interested, vain, and hypocritical politicians and rulers, who embrace noble causes only when these can be made to serve personal ambition or vanity.

Ideas and ideals by themselves do not impel action unless they are energized by emotion—especially by emotions awakened through conflict with opposing ideas and conditions. We could not struggle for justice or for the recognition of merit if injustice, hypocrisy, and imposture did not wound us deeply, threatening the very foundations of our existence. The intellectually superior individual, being less directly vulnerable to injustice than the emotionally or practically oriented person, is therefore rarely a leader in the passionate struggle for justice, love, merit, and true solidarity.

Under the present rule of hypocrites, parasites, masked criminals, and flatterers who appear as servants while acting as masters, the noble-minded are condemned to lives of renunciation and self-denial. Material well-being demands too high a price from honest individuals. Whoever seeks bodily comfort must often pay with the integrity of his own soul. One cannot serve two masters—especially when those masters, material success and self-perfection, are in open conflict.

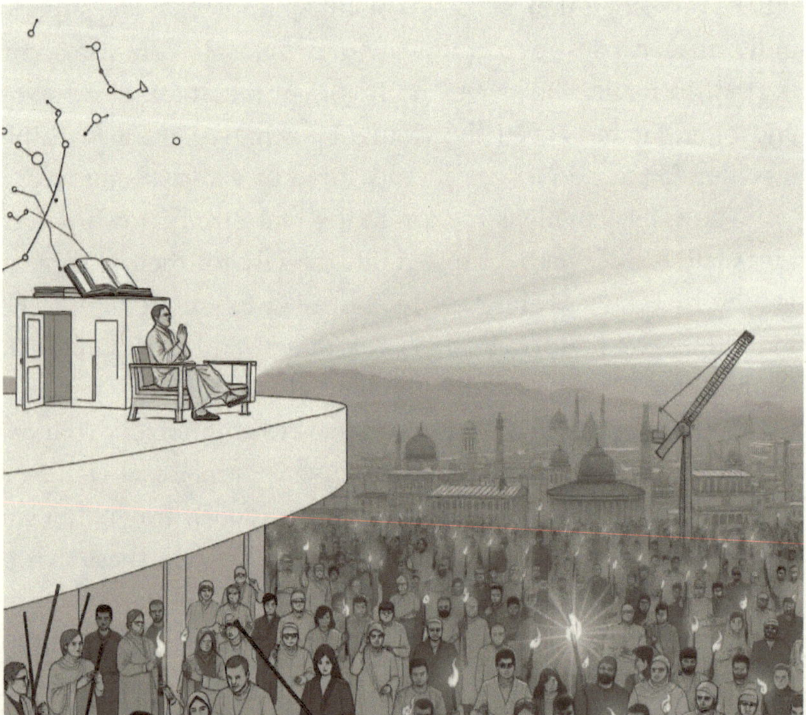

In a world where sham merit reigns supreme, it is easy to understand why the natural desire for social recognition and approval has lost its place, for the ideal individual, as a primary aim of life. It no longer functions as a motive or driving cause of action, but only as an accidental consequence—a secondary outcome that may or may not follow, but which no longer governs the direction of his striving. In emotionally superior individuals—in reformers, statesmen, and men of action—ideals exist more in the subconscious than in clear consciousness. Their ideals are intertwined with the deepest layers of their emotional life, and from this fusion arises their unshakable energy. In intellectually superior individuals, by contrast, ideals must pass from the vast domain of the subconscious through the narrow gate of consciousness. In this transition, the original ideo-emotional complexes are inevitably broken apart; some of their associative force is lost. This is the source of the thinker's lesser practical effectiveness when compared with the reformer.

The reformer instinctively rejects skepticism. The thinker, however, welcomes skepticism as a valuable assistant—only to find, in many cases, that it ultimately dominates him and paralyzes action. A certain measure of skepticism is useful for analysis, but its dissolving power becomes harmful when it undermines the emotional syntheses that prepare for action. The reformer's ideals are not as elevated as those of the pure thinker, but they are more warmly colored, more earthbound, and more closely connected with the ideals of ordinary people and daily life. For this reason, they possess an irresistible urgency and an imperious demand for realization. The thinker acts upon men of action, and through them, indirectly, upon the masses.

The thinker may successfully combat scientific prejudices, yet he lacks the emotional force required to overcome social prejudices and to liberate humanity from primitive ideas and from obsolete, burdensome social institutions. It is less dangerous—though no more hopeful—for the polemicist to champion scientific freedom from prejudice. Prejudice, in its broadest sense, is unavoidable and even useful, since it represents the judging of present experiences in the light of accumulated past experience. What must be resisted is not prejudice itself, but its tyranny. Prejudgment should serve as a preparatory stage of thinking, not as its permanent substitute.

Observation and interpretation, imitation and creation, consciousness and self-consciousness, thinking and acting, cannot exist with equal intensity at the same time. The curve of one lags almost ninety degrees behind the curve of the other. Maximum observation and thinking coincide with minimum action, and conversely. This explains why thinkers are relatively inactive during the rising phase of their intellectual development and become more active only after maturity or stagnation is reached. Men of action, on the other hand, often turn to pure thought once their practical goals have been achieved. What holds true for individual processes also holds true for individual and social life as a whole. Thinking and acting, contemplation and striving, are successive phases of a single circuit.

Moreover, the thinker's mind contains many parallel circuits at once—multiple streams of thought operating simultaneously. This further retards outward activity. The pure man of action, by contrast, concentrates his energy on realizing a single line of ideas and therefore acts swiftly and with great intensity. The thinker's energy is divided among many converging or diverging lines of thought. When these lines diverge, his action is prompt but weak; when they converge, it is powerful but delayed. The genuine and honest superior individual may become a man of action later in life, after forming stable, workable convictions.

The born man of action—the ambitious leader or pseudo-superior individual—becomes active in early life, before possessing any convictions of his own. He adopts the ideas of others only so long as they serve his personal interests. The pseudo-superior individual, unlike the genuine superior one, never forgets to display himself even in the midst of his most passionate speeches. He ensures that his audience never loses sight of his personality and never becomes wholly absorbed in the impersonal ideas he claims to defend.

True martyrs are rarely found among men of genius. Whether this is because martyrdom stirs emotion without promoting understanding, because the genius cannot sacrifice himself to a single idea when he is capable of many, or because he perceives the inadequacy of martyrdom as a means of enlightenment, the result remains the same. Martyrs are usually narrow in ideas and excessive in emotion; they overestimate the value of their convictions and underestimate the limits of sacrifice as a tool of progress. Religious and patriotic fanatics, moreover, have been taught to value earthly life lightly, having been conditioned to view death as a gateway to eternal reward.

Aims and Activity

The philistine is intellectually indolent. Ready-made opinions, dogmas, prejudices, borrowed feelings, and foreign initiative therefore appeal to him. The genius, on the other hand, is often physically indolent. He prefers to leave bodily labor—food, shelter, clothing, and comfort—to others. Yet both types are honest and consistent, each willing to exchange services and to limit claims to the fruits of the other's labor. The philistine is content with gossip, sensation, and superficial knowledge; the genius willingly renounces comfort and luxury if his abilities do not bring material reward.

Between these two stands the dishonest intermediary: the pseudo-superior individual. He poses as an intellectual producer when dealing with philistines and as an economic producer when dealing with geniuses. He buys and sells the labor and creations of both, robs the genius of recognition, and deprives the masses of the material goods they produce. He never exerts mental or physical effort for its own sake, but only when personal gain is assured.

The average person strives to please, to imitate, and to conform to public opinion, which represents a collective image of the ideal citizen and the ideal society. The superior individual strives to act according to an inner ideal—one that does not destroy public opinion but completes it. The ordinary person accepts the world as it is; the superior individual seeks to transform it, not to overthrow it. He shapes public opinion more than he is shaped by it.

The intellectual genius seeks truth; the emotional genius seeks beauty; the practical genius seeks utility; the moral genius seeks social happiness. One-sided superiority tends to sacrifice all other aims to the one pursued. Any sincere aim exerts not only a guiding but an energizing force, either by concentrating scattered abilities or by withdrawing energy from other pursuits. Laziness, apathy, or timidity do not always indicate weakness; they may arise from ignorance of one's own powers or from the absence of meaningful aims and outlets. Inactivity is the exception in the universe; activity is the rule. To live—to exist—is to act.

Conversely, displays of courage and energy are not always signs of strength. They may rest on the weakness of others or on the consuming intensity of a particular aim. Even timid animals show extraordinary courage when defending their young. The moral genius, despite poverty, obscurity, weakness, and isolation, dares to confront entrenched prejudices and expose hidden crimes of the powerful because moral elevation is the irresistible purpose of his life. He persists not because he denies human evil, but because he understands that most wrongdoing arises not from pleasure in cruelty, but from social conditions that offer no other means of satisfying human desires.

Greed emboldens the miser to defy contempt and danger. Vanity has transformed many trembling men into celebrated heroes. The credulity of the masses and the silent self-interest of followers have preserved such illusions. Even despair can momentarily turn the timid into the brave. Love, danger, or necessity can awaken energy where none seemed to exist.

If pseudo-superior individuals appear more energetic than genuine superior ones in defending noble causes, it is because such causes merely conceal selfish aims. If the thinker appears less active than the philistine, it is because his activity belongs to another order. His labor is inward rather than outward, mental rather than muscular, directed toward the shaping of ideas rather than the conquest of appearances.

When the genuine superior individual avoids popularity, it is not because he is entirely free from vanity. Rather, he knows—or instinctively feels—that the admired man, the idol of the intellectually blind masses, is forced to live on the surface of himself. The person whose exterior is constantly scrutinized, whose words are eagerly consumed, whose gestures are imitated, and whose actions are ceaselessly watched must inevitably neglect introspection and self-examination. He is drawn away from inner concentration, from lofty, impersonal, disinterested, and impartial thought, and compelled to descend into the lower realm of appearances, self-complacency, and petty personal concerns. He must emphasize, display, and exaggerate the quantitative, superficial, and eye-catching elements of his personality, sacrificing the qualitative, inward, deeper, and invisible aspects that are far more significant.

Man is, by nature, a being who strives upward and forward. When this striving is blocked—whether by incapacity or by external barriers—he does not simply remain at the level of basic animal pursuits such as food, shelter, and reproduction. Instead, he degenerates. Excess energy is then spent in exaggerated indulgence of these elementary pursuits: gluttony, luxury, ostentatious display, sensuality, compulsive accumulation, rapacity, aimless travel, and restless wandering. A particularly grotesque image of such degeneration appears in the parasitic dependents of the wealthy classes—figures morally and intellectually crippled, absorbed solely in the exhibition of wealth, the pursuit of selfish pleasures, and the maintenance of physical attractiveness as a means of power over others.

Because human beings must always hope for or strive toward something higher, they will pursue even illusory or spurious distant goals rather than none at all. They will idealize inferior aims—aims they would otherwise disregard—if no nobler purpose is offered to them. Thus we see the enthusiastic sons of aristocrats and industrial exploiters loudly embracing the cause of oppressed peasants and workers—whom they neither understand nor truly value—only to exploit them later in life when personal interests demand it. In the same way, young men from privileged classes who once fought passionately for emancipation did so not from deep concern for injustice, but from a lack of higher aims. Had they truly cared, they would not have been satisfied with granting a hollow freedom that merely replaced one form of bondage with another.

The pseudo-superior individual is too materialistic to devote time and patience to higher, non-remunerative pursuits. Yet the inborn impulse to aspire forces him to deceive himself by idealizing his selfish aims, or by persuading himself and others that these aims are merely accidental means toward higher, spiritual ends. The philistine unconsciously longs for friendship, justice, general happiness, beauty, and deeper insight into life. But his inability to attain or appreciate these genuine values leads him to idealize their empty imitations. What he calls friendship is often mutual exploitation disguised as mutual service; a telling example is the ritual exchange of gifts intended to secure future advantage. What he calls education or charity is frequently ostentation, ritual, or self-glorification. What he calls religion is superstition; patriotism becomes blind idolization and hostility toward outsiders; conversation becomes gossip; monogamy becomes concealed multiplicity, reduced at best to bodily restraint.

Unable to strive for authentic love, knowledge, beauty, altruism, or self-perfection, the philistine welcomes the pseudo-superior individual, who spares him effort by supplying ready-made imitations and sustaining the illusion of genuine possession. Incapable of drawing inspiration from distant futures envisioned by ideal thinkers, he prefers the false promises and immediate hopes offered by pseudo-superior figures. To abandon striving altogether is impossible, for the instinct to aspire cannot be extinguished. Even the flight of workers from monotonous labor to crude entertainments and gambling reflects this need—an attempt to discharge aspiration where no higher outlet is accessible or permitted.

Reward for Right Action

To work under the impulse of enduring influence or lasting recognition brings a reward as real as material success. Even when recognition is postponed to the future, belief in its eventual realization sustains life through sacrifice and renunciation. Human beings derive joy not only from attainment but from hope itself, and even from the means employed in pursuit of a goal. One cannot gain the admiration of distant places, future generations, or discerning minds without renouncing the approval of immediate surroundings and contemporary crowds. Ideal pursuit and worldly success are incompatible aims. If an ideal individual attains both during his lifetime, it is not because his ideals are understood, but because of accidental advantages such as wealth, position, or inherited rank. When the superior individual seeks wealth, it is not from servitude to desire, but because wealth signifies independence, and independence is a condition of self-perfection.

The materialist and the idealist both act logically, but from different premises. What appears rational from one standpoint appears meaningless from the other. The guiding axiom of the self-seeker is: Do whatever leads to your success. Its corollary is the need to please those who control advancement and to magnify one's own role. The axiom of the ideal individual is: Do whatever leads to truth, beauty, general happiness, or morality. Its corollary is the suppression of fame and material gain whenever these threaten higher aims.

From the perspective of enduring meaning, ideas and values are more real than fleeting individuals and sensations. From the perspective of immediate existence alone, the reverse seems true. Each standpoint is coherent within its own limits.

Leadership

Experience suggests that leadership often arises less from strength of character than from its absence. It is more frequently rooted in diminished moral restraint, weakened sincerity, and reduced altruism than in surplus energy or wisdom. Vanity and ambition, masked as insight, often replace genuine conviction. This is especially true of leaders who impose themselves without being needed, for whom no social necessity has prepared the ground. As history repeatedly shows, the world is often governed with remarkably little true wisdom.

Leaders, organizers, and politicians of this type are often innately immoral or amoral.

They live lives of moral duplicity, guided by two distinct moral codes: one private and sealed, the other public and constantly displayed.

They act morally or immorally according to the demands of personal or party interest. For them, morality is not an end, not a living force or inner aspiration, but merely a means—a convenient idea. Moral conduct may appear in their actions, yet it does not originate in their feelings or intentions. Their morality proceeds from calculation, not from instinct.

Some possess a natural gift for physiological mimicry—faces that appear harmless, innocent, or benevolent. Others display linguistic and mental mimicry: the ability to conceal cruelty, falsehood, and egotism behind a rich supply of memorized phrases, smooth gestures, and pleasing expressions; the ability to verbally appropriate the opinions, sentiments, and aspirations of others. For this reason, verbal fluency and easy command of sentimental language should be regarded with suspicion in moral diagnosis. Genuine feeling does not readily find such polished and convenient expressions. Oratorical skill is often both a cause and a result of moral and intellectual superficiality. Why labor to think deeply or act originally if combinations of words can simulate originality and verbal abundance can conceal inner poverty? Why cultivate noble thoughts or restrain base impulses when it is easier to adopt the language and manners of those who live nobly, while continuing prosaic pursuits under exalted names?

Figures such as Jesus, Buddha, Confucius, Moses, and Karl Marx do not fall under this rule. Yet even of such ideal leaders it may be said that they did not fully realize their potential idealism. Their actual individuality remained below their possible individuality because they were compelled to act directly upon the confused emotions and undeveloped ideas of intellectually blind masses. Even the morality—paradoxical though it may sound—of leaders in ethical or social movements, while superior to that of other political figures, is often inferior to the morality of their simplest followers.

It is therefore not surprising that the masses are so easily misled by demagogues, social quacks, and pseudo-leaders. After countless ages of slavery, exploitation, oppression, and the systematic destruction of independent and self-respecting individuals and peoples, the working masses consist largely of men and women brutalized by dependence and insecurity, crippled by oppression, and absorbed by immediate material needs. They are thus ill-prepared to respond to the personal influence of moral geniuses—individuals who look far into the future, whose enthusiasm is invested in ultimate aims rather than immediate gains, who appeal to reason rather than blind emotion, and who refuse to flatter the masses without also reproaching them for servility, lack of self-respect, and submissive acceptance of degrading conditions.

Though the moral genius believes in the eventual regeneration of humanity through the working masses—because of their moral superiority over unproductive classes—he cannot ignore their degradation nor praise virtues they do not yet possess, as the demagogue does. Nor can he accept the comforting illusion that popular ignorance and inferiority are due solely to lack of opportunity and will disappear automatically with economic improvement. He takes his mission too seriously and too disinterestedly to compromise, to flatter, to make empty promises, or to tolerate insincere, mercenary, or vain collaborators. He is too deeply concerned with the welfare of the human species—present and future—to confine his devotion to a small circle of followers in order to secure popularity. He is too frank and uncompromising to earn the tolerance of those who profit from predatory systems. His open contempt for entrenched power and privileged corruption inevitably provokes persecution against any movement he directly leads.

Pursuit of Truth and Struggle for Existence

Just as suicide, alcoholism, servility, flattery, and resignation are negative responses to the struggle for material or emotional security—signs of exhaustion rather than strength—so in the pursuit of truth, exaggerated mysticism, obscure transcendentalism, contempt for logic and reason, and the sentimental glorification of instinct or intuition are often symptoms of intellectual retreat rather than advance. At best, they represent negative paths toward truth.

Obscure and abstract writing, when practiced half-consciously, reveals not only a confused and chaotic mind but also a desire to impress the unthinking masses, to overawe public opinion, and to gain credit for meanings never clearly expressed but unconsciously supplied by the reader.

The essential difference between the striving life of the genuinely balanced superior individual and that of the ordinary or pseudo-superior individual lies here: the former subordinates personal interest, vanity, and self-love to truth; the latter subordinates truth to personal advantage. What is an organic necessity and commanding aim for the former becomes a luxury or a tool for the latter.

Among pseudo-superior individuals, two extreme types may be distinguished. The more intellectual type, in whom vanity outweighs materialism, often enters liberal professions—education, journalism, law, or ecclesiastical careers—forms of indirect parasitism. The less intellectual type, in whom materialism predominates and whose physical traits emphasize appetite and force, gravitates toward political, commercial, administrative, speculative, or technical pursuits—forms of direct parasitism. Between these extremes lie many intermediate forms, indifferent to social status so long as profit is assured.

The genuine superior individual does not deliberately sell or prostitute his intellectual gifts. He keeps his vocation distinct from his means of livelihood. He possesses little talent for profit, lacking the immoral skill required to exploit his own abilities—still less those of others. The pseudo-superior individual—the parasite masquerading as a benefactor—lives by exploiting ungrounded fears and empty hopes, poverty and ignorance, superstition and illusion, prejudice and antipathy; in short, by feeding upon the weaknesses of the masses. The genuinely superior individual, by contrast, appeals to their strength: to their productive capacity, latent abilities, realizable hopes, teachability, and nobler potential selves.

The pseudo-superior individual rules through force and coercion—through violence, persecution, and terror; by threats, intimidation, confusion, and intellectual stupefaction; by deceit, intrigue, fraud, imposture, and false promises; by intensifying fear, anxiety, and discord; by spreading unjustified alarm; by belittling the people's capacities while exaggerating his own supposed wisdom or resourcefulness; by diverting attention toward fictitious dangers and away from real ones.

The genuine superior individual seeks to lead through love and persuasion: by enlightening, encouraging, and consulting the people; by awakening dissatisfaction with the present while nurturing hope for the future; by fostering self-confidence and voluntary, intelligent cooperation; by dispelling discord and paralyzing fears; by identifying real yet removable dangers and their causes; by modestly acknowledging his own limitations and his merely advisory role; by inviting criticism, cooperation, and public oversight; and by urging the people to develop their dormant powers of self-rule, self-education, and self-help.

When the pseudo-superior individual exploits the hopeful side of human nature, he does so in a way that exhausts and stupefies his victims through excessive excitement, driving them inevitably toward the opposite extreme—fear, anxiety, despondency—where they fall prey to another exploiter who thrives on dread of illness, death, the future, accidents, the unknown, and life itself. Thus, the merchants of optimism and pessimism support one another. Even when the pseudo-superior individual adopts enlightenment or social reform as a profession, he combats ignorance and social evils only superficially and verbally—half-heartedly, playfully, and with ulterior motives—often remaining a secret accomplice of those who perpetuate ignorance, fear, misery, and servitude. By contrast, when the genuine superior individual calls the people to serious effort, he welcomes humor and recreation only insofar as they refresh the mind intelligently; and when he confronts wrongdoing and wrongdoers, he does so seriously, disinterestedly, thoroughly, uncompromisingly, and with full commitment.

Few writers have exposed the concealed predatory structure of modern society as powerfully as Upton Sinclair in The Jungle. The spirit and methods of the jungle persist, thinly disguised, within human society—maintained by predatory and would-be aristocratic philistines in general, and by pseudo-superior individuals in particular. Under the banners of business, promotion, leadership, philanthropy, religion, spiritual guidance, missionary zeal, and official science, these parasites continue their work of despoiling the masses or of assisting, directly or indirectly, in that process. Like wolves, they hunt in packs—gangs, cliques, and exclusive circles—where predatory philistines perform the menial tasks while pseudo-superior figures assume command. Outwardly, these groups appear devoted to the common good and harmonious cooperation; inwardly, they suffocate moral life through refined blackmail, intimidation, distrust, flattery, bluffing, and constant cowardly conflict over spoils and honors.

The exploiters understand well that their most dangerous enemies are living moral creators and revolutionaries—whatever names they bear. From the viewpoint of the predatory classes and their servants, distinctions among revolutionaries matter little, for all seek to abolish the jungle spirit and its methods, regardless of disguise. Indeed, exploiters often prefer to see reformers divided, quarreling over methods, rather than united in purpose.

The suspicion sometimes shown by working-class revolutionaries toward so-called "intellectuals" is not wholly unjustified, nor is it merely hostility toward education. Every genuine revolutionary is himself an intellectual in the truest sense, even without academic credentials or formal schooling. What he resists is the intrusion of self-seeking "intellectuals" who enter revolutionary movements to advance personal ambition after failing to secure positions among the retainers of capital or among professional flatterers.

The genuine superior individual is too absorbed in continuous learning and in thinking through new problems to interrupt his work, as the pseudo-superior does, to inventory his knowledge or measure his superiority over others. The more he reflects, the more perspectives unfold; the richer his inner world becomes, the more compelling new questions arise. Intellectual work is for him a source of deep enjoyment—an end in itself, not merely a means to status or self-display. Consequently, it never occurs to him to regard himself as intellectually "rich enough" to justify idleness or complacency.

The Lonely Path of Truth: Genius, Freedom, and the Future of Human Happiness

The apostle of truth, in his innocence, imagines that the masses are tormented by the same thirst for light and clarity that consumes him. He cannot conceive how human beings can live contentedly in the darkness of ignorance or in the dim twilight of illusion. Only when his efforts to awaken in others a love of truth are met with indifference, mockery, or silence does he begin to understand that the organ of truth is undeveloped or atrophied—not only in the ignorant and the emotional, but equally in the hunters of success, in philistines, pseudo-intellectuals, women, children, and immature or confused minds. Yet neither ingratitude nor derision can deter the true apostle of truth and love from his struggle against error, ignorance, falsehood, and evil.

Behind his abstract ideas, behind creations that appear impersonal, there stands—hidden from others but fully present to himself—the concrete, feeling personality of the thinker. Each abstract thought is the result of distillation, extracted from a vast accumulation of experience interwoven with personal joy and suffering. He might therefore fittingly preface his thoughts with these lines:

In these thoughts, however general and impersonal they may seem, lies buried a piece of my life, much hope, longing, and also tears.

It is in the nature of genius to express only what it recognizes as true, beautiful, and socially valuable, without regard for the harmful consequences this may bring to personal interest or to powerful institutions and classes. Genius and intellectual prostitution are incompatible. The expressions of genius are irrepressible and incorruptible. Communication may be postponed, but distortion, adulteration, or suppression is impossible.

When a creative individual appears to prostitute his intellectual individuality in order to safeguard personal interests, the appearance is deceptive. A starving genius may temporarily sacrifice a portion of his intellectual independence to preserve the minimum material conditions necessary for the survival and growth of his higher self.

If anyone may rightfully claim exemption from the struggle for mere subsistence, it is the man of genius, whose creations arise spontaneously and unpredictably and cannot be scheduled or postponed like the deliberate work of talent. Yet when forced to earn his livelihood, and given the choice between an occupation that demands sustained intellectual attention unrelated to his inner calling and one that is mechanical and automatic, he should choose the latter. Mechanical labor interferes less with spontaneous creation and allows the natural flow of thought to continue undisturbed. The genius is unfit for prolonged routine or narrowly specialized intellectual labor, for every external stimulus may awaken new, compelling trains of thought that it would be a tragedy to repress for the sake of unpromising routine.

To act under command means to inhibit one's own impulses, wishes, and spontaneity. Such inhibition is painful, especially when imposed from without or enforced by fear. Submissiveness is therefore easy for the empty-minded, the thoughtless, and the suggestible, but it is torture for the independent and creative mind. Demagogues succeed as commanders largely because their commands coincide with the impulses and desires of the masses. The ordinary man of action, who seeks activity as a narcotic, as proof of power, or as protection against inward reflection, readily surrenders his convictions—if he has any—and embraces any cause that allows free outward activity. The thinker and poet, by contrast, prefer to discipline the body in order to preserve the freedom of thought. They choose mechanical labor over intellectual work that contradicts their inner necessity, because such labor demands little attention and leaves the psyche free.

Originality and independent thought are natural gifts that endanger their possessor by making him conspicuous to tradition-bound masses and to those in power who fear intelligence. This explains why geniuses often avoid close social contact or disguise their originality by attributing it to divine inspiration, revelation, or tradition, or by masking it as eccentricity, humor, or even madness—forms that provoke ridicule or mild persecution rather than the lethal hostility that undisguised superiority arouses.

Pursuit of Social Happiness.—Motion is the primary and natural state of atoms, while rest characterizes bodies. Likewise, in simple organisms, spontaneous variation is fundamental, while stability is secondary. In higher organisms, physical stability becomes the rule, while mental variation remains rare and is confined to the small minority of geniuses. Mobility and progress are instinctive for intellectually developed individuals, who remain isolated; stagnation and routine suit the compact, unintellectual masses. Civilized societies, organized atomistically, progress rapidly but sacrifice equality and cohesion; primitive societies progress slowly but preserve solidarity and security.

The task of future moral genius—of mature socialism—will be to reconcile these opposites: progress with solidarity, liberty with security, individual creativity with cooperation, mobility with rootedness. Only through such synthesis can general social happiness be achieved. Communism, which differs fundamentally from modern socialism, has failed in complex societies not because it lacks moral intent, but because it is incompatible with liberty, intellectual development, and the higher forms of human fulfillment.

The moral genius declares war not only upon extra-social criminals—those who expiate their offenses through dishonor, restless wandering, and a life without peace—but even more decisively upon intra-social criminals: the pseudo-intellectual, pseudo-moral, and pseudo-religious individuals who never come into conflict with the law because they never violate its letter, while continually betraying its spirit. These individuals enjoy all the advantages of civilized society; they reap honor, fame, and wealth while living at the expense of genuine intellectual, moral, and religious workers. They discourage and enslave those who strive honestly; they trample upon the most sacred sentiments, aspirations, and convictions; they drive the helpless and friendless toward vagabondage, and the intellectually and morally impoverished toward extra-social crime. The moral genius therefore wages war against impostors disguised as saints, against idlers masquerading as busy men, against exploiters cloaked as benefactors, against anarchists hiding behind the role of lawmakers and guardians of order. His struggle is directed less against institutions as such than against their imperfections; less against parasites in the form of beggars and tramps—whom society supports from its surplus—than against parasites in the form of aristocrats, capitalists, and speculators who, indirectly but relentlessly, compel society to feed and enrich them while starving its own minds and bodies. He fights not so much the parasites themselves as the circumstances and institutions that permit or compel parasitism; not the visible effects, but the deep-rooted causes of social evil.

In his constructive work, the moral genius takes—more or less consciously—the relationships within an ideal family as the prototype for relationships within an ideal society. Such relations are founded not on written statutes and printed stipulations, nor on formal justice and mechanical equality, but on living sentiments of love and solidarity impressed upon the heart of every member. Each person holds the rank he deserves, works according to ability, and is provided for according to need. Without the recurring, renewing influence of moral geniuses upon language, customs, and institutions—academic ones included—these structures decay into lifeless mechanisms, empty routines, and obstacles to progress. They harden into red tape, that dangerous social gangrene which spreads through the social organism and would ultimately destroy it, were it not for the timely warning and remedies applied by social physicians—the moral geniuses.

The moral genius senses, whether consciously or not, that the only truly valuable building blocks of a just and solidary society are the hard-working, honestly striving, obscure and unobtrusive individuals, together with those superior minds who attain recognition without seeking it. He recognizes as useless—and indeed dangerous—financial speculators, sham aristocrats, and intra-social criminals: individuals congenitally greedy, narrow-hearted, insatiable, and parasitical, whose intelligence is consumed entirely in devising methods for enslaving others and robbing them under the pretense of service. Their sole talent lies in exploiting the ignorance, helplessness, poverty, and trust of others; in shifting the burdens and risks of life onto the shoulders of the uninformed and the poor.

Moral geniuses and social reformers have therefore always gravitated, in one form or another, toward cooperation or socialism. They have foreseen—dimly or clearly—that if all services rendered to individuals were recognized as services rendered to the community, and were therefore regulated and remunerated by the community itself, according to real needs and capacities, many social distortions would disappear. Services would be valued by competent specialists rather than by ignorant or incapable recipients, as occurs in an unregulated, competitive society. There would be no persistent gap between ability and success, no space for cunning charlatans and demagogues to thrive at the expense of naïve clients or voters.

Under such conditions, fulfilling one's duty and earning social appreciation would no longer require two separate and often contradictory abilities; individuals would no longer be forced to split their convictions and morality into a private and a public code. To eliminate the arbitrary and uncertain remuneration of services by incompetent judgment; to correct the grotesque disproportions between supply and demand produced by unchecked competition and lack of wise regulation—this would remove the principal causes of soul-destroying economic dependence, favoritism, nepotism, greed, corruption, charlatanism, and the waste of human time and energy in purely material pursuits. It would curb tyranny and slavery, and prevent the pathological proliferation of unnecessary parasitical professions that insert themselves between producers and consumers, draining the life of the social organism.

End of the Chapter

Chapter-7.
How Minds Are Moved:
Thought, Art, and the Shaping of the Masses

This chapter reveals the hidden mechanics by which ideas travel from solitary minds into collective life. It shows why artists move hearts faster than thinkers move reason, how suggestion often outweighs argument, and how genuine creators shape the masses indirectly—offering readers a deeper understanding of who truly influences society and why.

Influence of Thinkers and Artists

It is no mere metaphor to say that the ordinary individual cannot truly see with his own eyes – especially not with the mind's eye. He sees and acts largely in response to what geniuses suggest to him. The poet stirs and impels to action; the thinker guides and opens vast horizons; the man of action leads. We do not perceive new objects, relations, or meanings until intellectual creators have prepared our minds to receive them. In the same way, we do not feel genuine love or obligation toward other classes, nations, or races until moral creators have planted these sentiments in our hearts.

Just as we instinctively close our physical eyes when passing abruptly from darkness into bright light, because the pain allows no time for adjustment, so we close the eyes of the mind when suddenly confronted with truth after long immersion in ignorance or illusion. Such a transition is painful, for the intellect and the emotions need time to adapt to new light.

Progress is of little value if each advance is preceded or followed by a retreat. Without preservation, there can be no lasting progress. Jurisprudence, legislation, and the state are primarily concerned with conservation—with maintaining an existing moral level and equilibrium. Ethics, on the other hand, seeks to raise that level. The former represents moral statics, the latter moral dynamics. Jurisprudence requires acts and facts; ethics requires intentions. The former aims to make people less dangerous; the latter to make them more useful and better. Jurisprudence is thus a negative form of ethics.

Beyond morality, however, lies a broader domain: sympathy. This wider sphere includes morality but also extends beyond it. Morality concerns intentional acts and the accompanying sense of responsibility. An expanded ethical vision would also encompass unintentional acts and their social consequences, together with feelings of moral satisfaction or regret. The sphere of sympathy goes still further, embracing social events that are not decisively shaped by any single individual. A creator who influences this realm of sympathy therefore fulfills a higher function than one who acts solely within the narrower moral domain.

Form is more accessible to the majority than essence. Form first appeals to the senses, while essence appeals to reason. This explains why artists, poets, and orators exert a broader and more immediate influence over the masses than thinkers, scientists, or philosophers. Thinkers affect the masses indirectly, through the mediation of emotional and active individuals.

The wider social and cultural environment acts upon the mind of the superior individual. In turn, the genuine superior individual influences others quietly and disinterestedly—often even to his own disadvantage—through his works and writings. These reach the book-reading public and the vain, semi-materialistic pseudo-superior individuals, who then transmit diluted versions of these ideas to the non-reading masses. This occurs either directly, through speech and personal influence, or indirectly through newspapers and magazines.

If we move from the non-reading public to newspaper readers, from these to magazine readers, and finally to book readers, we observe a gradual widening of intellectual horizon and a corresponding transformation of interests. What begins as local, superficial, personal, and self-interested gradually becomes universal, deeper, impersonal, and disinterested. The thinker's preference for books over newspapers and magazines arises not only from the triviality of much of their content, but above all from the fact that even this content is often distorted in the service of private or class interests.

The philistine is largely impervious to the subtle, intangible influence of ideas unless these ideas are associated with a person of visible prestige—someone he can see, hear, or recognize. The magazine or novel reader, who stands somewhat higher intellectually, is more sensitive to abstract influence, yet even he usually requires reinforcement through the perceived presence or authority of a living author. Purely depersonalized scientific or philosophical ideas—detached from the voice of an orator, from the prestige of a known personality, from personal obligations, and from the concealed interests served by popular media—reach and influence only the highly sensitive intellect of the genuine thinker.

Thinkers need not lament their limited direct influence. This apparent disadvantage safeguards the purity of their thought. Rare indeed is the admired individual who does not become, consciously or unconsciously, the slave or flatterer of those who admire him. Moreover, fame, like wealth, attracts its own parasites. The prominent figure gradually becomes an unconscious flatterer of his admirers—not so much of those who originally admired him for his truth or originality, but of those who admire him out of imitation, fashion, or fear of appearing incapable of recognizing merit. Many admire success itself, without understanding the substance or value of what is admired.

Reason alone does not convince the masses; suggestion is what captures their attention. When a celebrated genius addresses the public, he may believe—naïvely—that understanding and agreement have been produced by his arguments. In reality, it is his personality and reputation that have created the response. The same words, spoken with equal or greater eloquence by an unknown individual, would have been ignored.

The mind of the genius, and of the genuinely superior individual, is elastic. When one system of ideas is drawn in a new direction, other systems that are closely or remotely connected are naturally pulled along with it. The movement spreads without tearing the fabric of thought. The mind of the philistine, by contrast, is inelastic, though to some extent malleable. New ways of thinking and acting must be slowly and patiently hammered in, while old habits must be hammered out through repeated suggestion. If compelled to accept sudden changes all at once, such a mind does not adapt—it breaks, and moral disintegration follows.

In an elastic mind, when a group of ideas expands or is redirected, its connections with other ideas are not destroyed; they merely rearrange themselves, while the harmony of the whole remains intact. In a rigid, dogmatic, custom-bound mind, however, pressure from new currents of thought causes the system to split into disconnected fragments. These fragments lose their anchorage and begin to drift aimlessly, like uprooted plants carried about by water and wind. This explains, in part, why the sudden and forced "civilizing" of primitive peoples so often results in demoralization: their natural mental elasticity is overstrained.

Yet the deeper cause of their degeneration and disappearance lies in the fact that they are usually brought into contact not with the best representatives of civilization, but with greedy adventurers and the moral refuse of so-called civilized nations. The needs of philistines—and especially of women, in this psychological sense—are often vague, ill-defined, and highly susceptible to suggestion. They are shaped less by inner or outer reality than by external influence. As a result, the philistine does not know how to recognize, let alone pursue, the objects capable of truly satisfying these needs. He therefore feels the necessity of a guide, a leader, a teacher who tells him what is valuable, what deserves attention, admiration, pursuit, pride, or aversion. He prefers a living person to a book or to nature itself. A book requires interpretation, and nature speaks only in hints; but from a living guide—through words, gestures, tone, and attitude—he can immediately sense what is to be sought, admired, feared, or rejected, without reflection.

Left to himself, the philistine has neither strong attachments nor strong aversions toward people, things, or ideas. Under guidance and suggestion, however, his naturally weak emotions can be inflamed into passions that appear irresistible. It is far easier to implant emotions than ideas in him, easier to suggest attachments to persons and objects than to principles and ideals, and easier still to excite enthusiasm for form rather than for essence.

It is simpler to rouse passion for activities such as games, spectacles, fights, wars, and similar excitements that offer immediate but fleeting—and often harmful—pleasure, than for pursuits that bring lasting, elevating, and useful satisfaction without immediate reward.

Influence of Mystics

Mystical writers appear to exert a stronger influence over the majority than clear thinkers because their writings tell everyone what they wish to hear. Meaning is not drawn from such writings; it is read into them. Even earnest and intelligent individuals may fall prey to obscure, semi-delirious language, believing it a duty to understand everyone—even those who do not understand themselves.

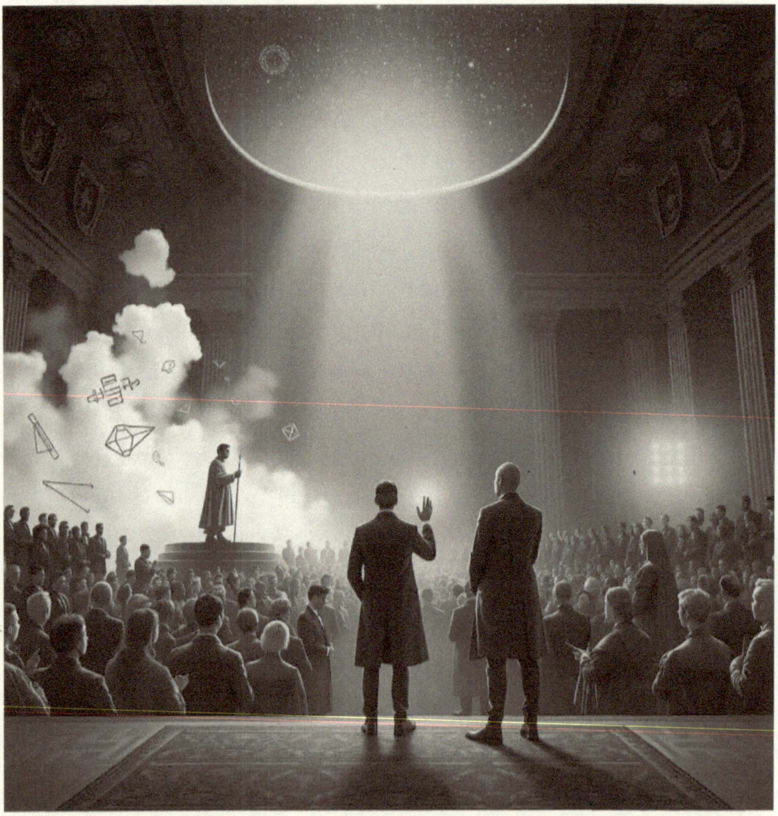

The mystic and pseudo-mystic apply abstract terms to concrete and trivial matters, creating the illusion of depth, originality, and lofty generalization where only commonplace thoughts exist. Otherwise their verbosity would be inexplicable, for one cannot speak endlessly without having something—however banal—in mind. The danger lies in the deceptive language, which obscures the true, often petty content beneath it. We imagine a lofty, impersonal, idealistic teacher, when in reality we face a sensual, materialistic, vain, personal, and resentful pseudo-superior individual.

The modern mystic—whether theologian, spiritist, or theosophist—pays superficial homage to science by adopting its vocabulary, at least in appearance. He is therefore mistaken for a scientist, despite lacking the discipline, skepticism, intellectual honesty, and devotion to truth that define genuine scientific thinking. The clear-minded, truth-loving thinker cannot attract large followings, because he expresses sharply defined views that compel either agreement or rejection. His precision leaves no room for evasive neutrality. By contrast, the nebulous, truth-avoiding thinker, uncertain even of his own position, spares readers the effort of ordering their thoughts. His language is misty and ambiguous; he shifts effortlessly between opposites, allowing each reader to find only what pleases him. No internal reorganization is demanded.

What the clear thinker accomplishes in the intellectual realm, the moral genius accomplishes in the social and economic sphere. He exposes the true motives behind human behavior. Those offended by his revelations are forced either to refute him through changed conduct or to accept the accusation by continuing their harmful practices.

Opposed to the moral genius stands the pseudo-moralist. Unlike the former, he makes no enemies. His denunciations of evil are so abstract and impersonal that no wrongdoer recognizes himself in them, and his defense of victims is weakened by subtle insinuations of their own fault. Thus, oppressors and oppressed alike nod in passive agreement.

The deliberately vague intellectual demagogue, like the political demagogue, presents himself as everyone's ally. Weak, insecure, fame-seeking pseudo-intellectuals gather around him for support once tradition and authority no longer suffice. He promises them protection, while in reality they sustain his reputation through their numbers. Should any of them grow suspicious when they notice that opponents also lean on him, he hastens to reassure them privately that they are his true favorites, while the others are merely tolerated. Thus we see intellectual opportunists of opposing camps cluster around a single philosophical demagogue, each believing himself uniquely favored, and none disturbed by the fact that irreconcilable enemies are welcomed with equal warmth.

In this way, ambiguity, not clarity; suggestion, not truth; and prestige, not understanding, become the dominant forces shaping the minds of the masses.

Why and How Far the Mass Is Influenced.—The majority of people live under the influence of extreme ideals. From the clash of these extremes arises a middle course, and it is this mean alone that proves strictly workable and useful in practice. Extreme views are the only ones that are logically consistent, but moderation is what life can actually sustain.

The influence exerted by superior individuals upon average men consists primarily in preparing their minds to view the world and human life in certain ways. It consists in placing the mind in a state of expectant attention toward the phenomena of nature and society. Before we are able to create, we must first imitate; and in order to imitate, we must already possess, at least unconsciously, a tendency in the same direction. The masses can imitate geniuses only because they carry within themselves, in germ, the same aspirations and capacities. They must be capable of resonance, of vibrating sympathetically in unison with the geniuses who arise among them. Conversely, the genius can influence the masses only if he strives along lines that correspond, at least in part, to the direction of the majority. Nature and society can be mastered only by obeying their laws.

We assimilate the ideas of others by means of our own ideas; we acquire the new through the old; we accomplish voluntarily what has its roots in spontaneous tendencies. Without some intellectual capital—however small—no intellectual enrichment is possible. Without such capital, the only alternative is to remain an intellectual laborer, thinking according to the patterns of intellectual capitalists, just as the financially poor must work according to the will of the financially rich. There is, however, a decisive difference—one that a more humane society may one day abolish—between the intellectual and the financial capitalist: the former does not exploit the intellectually poor; on the contrary, he places his intellectual capital at the service of all.

Helmholtz's theory, according to which we hear only those sounds and see only those colors whose vibrations find corresponding nerve fibers capable of sympathetic vibration, applies not merely metaphorically but quite literally to thought and understanding. We comprehend others, adopt their ideas, and share their feelings only insofar as our higher brain centers vibrate in sympathy with theirs. From the same books, speeches, dramas, or newspapers, people of different mental constitutions extract entirely different meanings. The good grow better, the bad more dangerous; the intelligent become clearer, the dull more confused. It is therefore meaningless to argue abstractly about the beneficial or harmful influence of books, education, religion, or doctrines. Daily life and history show clearly that no one can be permanently influenced to act against his nature and economic conditions; that verbal adherence to doctrines bears little relation to actual conduct; that under the same banner people fight for different motives and ends; and that preaching alone, without a transformation of the predatory and hierarchical foundations of society, has never abolished fundamental differences in human character. The real forces shaping the future of humanity are not professed doctrines, but the living influence exerted every day by productive and parasitical types of people upon one another and upon the large, plastic, impressionable mass of philistines.

Everyone learns from others what he wishes to learn, what aligns with his dominant interests. Every influential person hears from favorites and dependents exactly what he wishes to hear. If rulers, magnates, leaders, and celebrated figures are shielded from truth, it is not because truth cannot reach them, but because they do not desire it and do not encourage those who speak it.

The cognitive, emotional, and volitional geniuses influence the masses only insofar as they give clear and purposeful expression to the vague, hesitant, and unformed thoughts, feelings, and desires already present in the collective mind. Their inner states are more intense, more differentiated, and freer from the bonds of habit, fear, and unconscious inhibition. They are therefore better able to find expression in language, action, art, technique, and institutions.

To possess taste or critical ability is to recognize the adequacy of form—to welcome in others the expression of our own inner states which we either dare not express or cannot clearly articulate.

The critic, the interpreter, and the popularizer serve as intermediaries between the genius and the masses. The influence of poets is largely local and national; that of scientists and technologists is international; the influence of philosophers belongs more to the future than to the present. The lifespan of an intellectual work is inversely proportional to the number of people it directly influences. Artistic and literary works are the most fleeting; scientific works grow obsolete within decades; philosophical ideas alone approach immortality.

Why do average people—who live physically close yet remain mentally far apart—learn more about life from the stage than from real life, from poets rather than from actual heroes? First, because we identify ourselves with dramatic figures, and the sympathy we feel for them is in truth sympathy for ourselves. Second, because even characters unlike us speak openly and reveal their motives, allowing us deeper insight than we gain from real individuals. Third, because our personal interests do not clash with those of fictional figures, making sympathy easier.

Suggestion becomes effective only when it aligns with the will and the existing streams of consciousness of the person influenced. Suggested ideas must be introduced gradually into the mental current until, by accumulation, they redirect its flow without arousing resistance. In truth, no foreign will dominates here—the suggestion has become the individual's own.

Just as every physical action provokes an equal and opposite reaction, so every command provokes resistance—overt or suppressed—unless neutralized by fear or reinforced by love, admiration, confidence, or shared purpose. Hence a fundamental pedagogical rule, too often ignored: do not command or dogmatize until you have secured trust, respect, conviction, or goodwill.

In traditional and practical matters, even superior individuals fall under the suggestive influence of the masses, just as the masses fall under their influence in theoretical and innovative domains. No genius—especially a one-sided one—can permanently escape the rhythmic pressure of inheritance, education, tradition, and popular belief in areas outside his originality. Few geniuses succeed in freeing themselves entirely from the prejudices, false sympathies, and distorted values continually instilled by schools, churches, the press, and political platforms.

Suggestion, and especially hypnotic suggestion, differs fundamentally from logical persuasion. It deceives individuals into believing that they perceive, think, or desire what they do not. In social and political life it corresponds to the deceptive methods by which ambitious newcomers insinuate themselves into established elites. Sudden intrusion invites resistance; gradual, disguised entry succeeds when vigilance is dulled or attention diverted. The same logic governs psychological influence.

In a genuinely democratic society, where public life unfolds transparently and all have access to participation, such deceitful methods lose their power. Likewise, with broad-minded individuals who welcome ideas solely on their objective merit, hypnotic suggestion finds no foothold. Scientific and social education, unlike dogmatic and authoritarian systems, does not exploit immaturity and credulity. It does not rely on fear, mystification, or imposed beliefs beyond lived experience. Honest politics and an honest spiritual life require no secrecy, spectacle, or manipulation. They need only persuasion, enlightenment, and an appeal to the people's own interests, experience, and sense of justice.

How Suggestion Works.—The only difference between mechanical, physical, chemical, physiological, psychical, and social phenomena lies in their increasing degree of complexity. Attraction, gravitation, affinity, assimilation, love, and social solidarity are analogous processes of growing complexity, governed by the same fundamental law, though increasingly modified by the interference of other laws.

From a physical point of view, sympathy and antipathy may be reduced to processes of equalization between unequal degrees of similar emotional states. One who suffers less in a given respect sympathizes with another whom he imagines to suffer more in the same respect; one who enjoys less in a given respect may feel antipathy toward one who enjoys more in that same respect. The absence of sympathy—of emotional equalization—results from insulation or isolation. Thus, the capitalistic class, insulated within the sphere of industrial and selfish interests, fails to sympathize with the suffering of the poor, although individual members of that class may be or may become broad-hearted. Likewise, the class of average men, enclosed within the insulating medium of daily bodily needs, is inaccessible to the disinterested spiritual pursuits of men of genius, although the same individuals, when broken into smaller groups, can be readily reached by original and elevating ideas.

The emotional genius works through sympathetic equalization: he breaks down the insulating, dielectric barriers separating classes, nations, and races. The active genius breaks the insulating, misoneistic barrier between idea and act; he rubs off the psychical rust and incites action by acting himself.

The suggestive influence exerted by the genius upon the masses is analogous to the equalization of temperatures that occurs when a hot and a cold body are brought into contact. Just as such contact lowers the temperature of the hotter body and raises that of the colder, so contact between the genius and the masses lowers the genius and elevates the average man. In society, the genius simulates banality, and the average man simulates originality and loftiness of ideals—until this simulation becomes, in part, reality. Mental equalization begins with imitation but ends in conviction. Only the genius who refrains from acting directly upon the masses can permanently maintain himself at a high level.

Average men and pseudo-superior men stand, as individuals, on a lower plane than they do as members of society, public institutions, or organized opinion; superior men, on the contrary, stand higher as individuals than they do as members of collective bodies or as holders of public functions. Social, guild, and institutional life acts as a relentless leveling force. It raises the philistines and lowers the superior men who lack sufficient economic independence to influence society while remaining intellectually free. Such men often keep their distance from the professional or social groups nearest to them in order to preserve independence of judgment and freedom in the pursuit of truth. Woe to the genius who cannot, when irreconcilable conflict arises, sacrifice economic security, social solidarity, or even family affection to his stronger impulse toward the still solitary, uninhabited land of truth.

Within circles of intellectual men—scholars and thinkers—women learn to suppress or disguise their vain, impulsive, emotionally explosive natures and to simulate tolerance, reasonableness, calm reflection, and idealism.

It is exceedingly difficult to impose an original idea upon society, for no one dares to differ openly from the rest. Yet as soon as an original idea is favorably received by a few representatives of a social class, all other members hasten to profess it, for no one dares to lag behind. Thus the same force that makes social life an almost insurmountable obstacle to originality at its birth becomes, once the idea is endorsed by leaders, the most effective vehicle for its diffusion. Anti-parasitism or socialism advances slowly because the ruling classes, for obvious personal reasons, oppose it; whereas movements such as the Reformation or the Renaissance, which first gained the favor of rulers, spread rapidly among the masses. Suggestion operates by first diverting attention, then bringing into the foreground of consciousness what previously remained in the background. It aggregates mental states that were formerly disjointed and gives them the initial impulse toward action; once translated into action, it gives them direction. Retrograde suggestion works in the opposite manner: it transforms purposeful, regulated, serious activity into disoriented, chaotic, aimless, and playful movement. It reduces action to mere impulse or dissolves it into a system of empty ideas. Attention is first diverted from the guiding system of ideas, which is then gradually dissolved and disaggregated into the darkness of unconsciousness.

The suggestion exerted by geniuses, if it is to be effective, must operate from a distance and act intermittently. Geniuses always form a minority, and a minority can prevail over a majority only in two ways: indirectly, by acting from afar, creating the impression of being more numerous or more authoritative than it is; or directly, by attacking intermittently, briefly, and at different points, instead of engaging in continuous frontal contact. For this reason, geniuses usually exert little influence in the very places where they live in close, daily contact with the majority. In large cities, however, the mass of average individuals is broken up into many small groups, and these smaller units are far more accessible to the assault of original ideas.

Ideas of universal value gain momentum, authority, and compelling force in proportion to the spatial and temporal distance separating their originators from the masses upon whom they act. Contemporaries who live in immediate proximity to the masses rarely exercise a progressive influence over them. It is the dead who rule the living—not so much because of what they actually were or accomplished during their lifetime, but because their ideas and personalities have gained idealization, purification, authority, and accumulated prestige through the long distance of history and repeated transmission.

When a nation, a race, or a continent receives an impulse toward progress from another, this does not imply inferiority. It merely shows that the receiving society has less tolerance, respect, or receptivity for its own living geniuses than for distant or foreign ones. It shows that, alongside internal tendencies, an external impulse is often required to accelerate progress. There was a time when the Orient instructed Europe; later, Europe reacted upon Asia, which seemed to have lost its forward momentum. Such exchanges reveal not hierarchy, but differing phases of cultural and intellectual receptivity.

Living geniuses could never act efficiently or progressively upon the masses if they were not psychically isolated from them—if they were not sufficiently insulated to resist being drawn downward by the gravitational pull of the larger philistine mass. Their influence is possible only because the masses themselves, through the division of labor and social differentiation, are split into smaller, relatively isolated groups. These groups cannot unite their leveling forces against the creative minority and therefore become accessible, one after another, to elevating influences. Certain classes or circles are raised first to a higher intellectual or moral level; others follow later, and so on.

With increasing ease of travel and migration, intelligent, open-minded, and original individuals often leave the towns and countries where they lack prestige, courage, or suitable means to enlighten others. From a distance, from an adopted homeland, protected by anonymity or economic independence, their words gain authority and freedom. They can speak more openly, impartially, and safely to distant, personally unknown compatriots than to those who know them closely. Paradoxically, they are permitted to shed more light on remote places than on their immediate surroundings.

Between similar psychical elements—ideas with ideas, emotions with emotions—there exists mutual influence in the form of association, suggestion, and fusion. Between dissimilar elements—such as sensation and movement, imagination and action—the influence takes the form of induction. In both cases, however, intensity diminishes at the moment of transmission. A belief or conviction loses part of its force when it is communicated or put into practice, just as electrical pressure diminishes in a transformer when resistance is introduced into the circuit.

Thus, distance, isolation, and gradual transmission are not obstacles to influence; they are its very conditions. Only by withdrawing from the immediate pressure of the masses can the genius preserve the strength, clarity, and transformative power of his ideas—and only through distance can those ideas return with increased authority to reshape the minds of men.

End of the Chapter

Chapter-8.
Great Souls and Small Souls: The Tragedy of True Appreciation

This chapter exposes why true greatness is so often ignored while mediocrity is celebrated. It explores how small souls mistake noise for depth, fame for merit, and imitation for creation, revealing the tragic gap between genuine superiority and public recognition—and how readers can learn to see beyond appearances to real worth.

Difficulties in Appreciation

Our understanding and appreciation of things in the outer world develop in the same way as our understanding and appreciation of human beings in the inner world. Both progress gradually: from surface to depth, from what is near to what is distant, from what is changeable and fleeting to what is stable and enduring, from the loud and eye-catching to the quiet and unobtrusive, from brilliance that dazzles to truth that enlightens, from form to essence, from appearance to reality. In the same manner, our judgment moves from the superficial, self-advertising, noisy pseudo-superior individuals to the modest, inward, contemplative, self-effacing, genuinely superior men.

An uneducated fool or an obvious lunatic becomes an object of laughter even to children. By contrast, the incoherent speech of an educated borderline lunatic is often taken seriously—even by clear-minded thinkers—who then waste valuable time and mental energy attempting to extract meaning where none exists.

Small souls judge people by clothing, rank, or wealth, and ideas by their wording. Because deep thoughts remain obscure or unintelligible to them, they conclude that any mystical, confused, or grandiose language must conceal profound meaning. Hence their admiration for mystical writers—genuine or simulated—and their instinctive distrust or contempt for clear, lucid thinkers.

If language is the garment of thought, then it must fit what it clothes. A florid, dramatic, picturesque style may suit emotional expression, but it is ill-adapted to scientific or philosophical truth. Such truths possess a sublime simplicity and richness of content that no ornament can enhance. Decorative language only diverts attention away from the thought itself, consuming the reader's energy in images instead of insight. One day, philosophy expressed through metaphor and personification will appear as antiquated as science once expressed through mythology.

Pseudo-superior writers deliberately seek ornate, grandiloquent, or mystical language in order to distract from the banality—or emptiness—of the ideas beneath. In doing so, they attract admiration from readers who cannot imagine that genuine depth can exist behind clear, transparent, simple language. They resemble those who underestimate the depth of a river because its waters are so clear that the bottom is visible.

"No one is a prophet in his own land" because ordinary people unconsciously expect originality to manifest itself in every aspect of a superior person's existence—even in inherited traits, habits, or physiology. In doing so, they reveal their own lack of self-esteem: they expect the superior individual to be entirely unlike themselves in all respects.

To acknowledge merit in someone who can compel recognition through power, position, or prestige requires little honesty. Prudence and self-interest alone may dictate such acknowledgment, especially when dealing with ambitious, self-assertive individuals. It is easy to bow before established fame. But to discover genuine merit independently—or to dethrone false merit—demands critical courage, intellectual independence, and moral strength beyond the average.

This reluctance to expose impostors and to recognize authentic originality is especially marked among parasitical, self-appointed critics and among vain academicians and professors. They import into the intellectual sphere the aggressive competitiveness of the economic world and the narrow sectarian spirit of politics, replacing truth-seeking with rivalry, caste loyalty, and self-protection.

The value of average individuals lies chiefly in their physical strength or skill and in their capacity for organization and association. They shine not by their own light, but by reflecting the light of the groups to which they belong. They are satellites revolving around group leaders—who themselves revolve around distant, largely invisible geniuses. These geniuses are the solitary stars of humanity. Their intense light is at first perceptible only through the psychological telescopes of a select minority. Long after their extinction, that light finally reaches the unaided eyes of the great mass of ordinary men.

Thus the tragedy of appreciation unfolds: the shallow are admired quickly, loudly, and excessively, while the profound are misunderstood, ignored, or resisted—only to be recognized when distance, time, and purification have transformed their truth into authority.

The philistine constantly confuses the interpreter with the creator: the popularizer or journalist with the original thinker; the empty, pleasure-seeking fraternity student with the sincere seeker of knowledge; the performer with the composer; the reciter with the poet; the professor of philosophy with the philosopher; the lawgiver or ruler with the true originator of laws, the social reformer, the genuine benefactor of society; the flatterer or demagogue with a friend or altruist; the preacher with the moral genius; the gossiping writer with the novelist; the dealer in phrases with the original mind; the actor with the dramatist. In short, he mistakes pseudo-superior or self-styled semi-superior men for the genuinely superior individuals whom they merely imitate, echo, or imperfectly transmit, and whose inspirations they realize slowly, incompletely, and often unfaithfully.

This error of judgment arises because pseudo- and semi-superior men are closer to the philistine in temperament and outlook. Moreover, driven by vanity or material interest, they thrust themselves into public view, make themselves conspicuous, and appear intelligible to the masses.

It is remarkable that human beings—supposedly the most intelligent of animals—are often the least capable of distinguishing a genuine leader from an impostor. Instead of following the true leader, the one willing to stand in front, exposed to the greatest danger and hardship, they worship dignified-looking scoundrels: cowards masquerading as heroes, parasites posing as guides. These figures hide behind their followers, using them as shields against attack or as ladders to climb into secure, privileged, and unassailable positions. Human beings are the only animals who fight the battles of their leaders against rivals; other gregarious animals allow contenders for leadership to fight among themselves and then follow the victor—the strongest.

Negligible quantities are often overvalued when, by their addition, they disturb an equilibrium and tip the scales. In the same way, men of little talent and pseudo-superior individuals are overestimated when they attach themselves to lofty ideals already floating in the air and nearing realization. Whoever possesses the instinct to detect such movements and drift with the current not only gains the reputation of an idealist, but can also indulge grossly materialistic desires with impunity.

The pseudo-superior man hides his lack of noble feeling behind apparently altruistic actions, and conceals his unwillingness to act behind an excess of simulated sentiment. Beneath the mask of apparent calm, reflection, and gravity, he conceals frivolity, pettiness, and a cold, self-centered heart. Beneath a perpetually smiling, kindly expression, he hides a lack of true social feeling and genuine sympathy. This assumed gravity—often a refined form of the intimidating instinct found in animals—is also meant to frighten others into submission and respect.

In their judgments, the masses do not know how to distribute praise and criticism with balance. They either admire everything a superior person says or does—including faults, eccentricities, intellectual weeds, and half-insane acts—or they ridicule everything in him, even his most humane and fertile ideas and actions. They cannot proportion praise and blame within the same individual. They do not understand how a sound and superior mind may still be deficient or unbalanced in certain respects, or how a man superior to them may share many of their ordinary weaknesses. Instead, they prefer to interpret such weaknesses as mere appearances or as necessary companions of higher qualities.

The masses also confuse extremes, because they focus on superficial similarities. Thus, they mistake the insane for the genius and the genius for the insane, since both are original and deviate from the norm. They mistake nonsense for depth of thought, because both lie beyond their understanding. They fail to grasp that the originality of insanity arises from a deficiency of inhibition and a tyranny of vanity, whereas the originality of genius springs from a surplus of energy. They do not see that the obscurity of deep thought is due to its abstraction and breadth of vision, while the obscurity of nonsense results from incoherence and the absence of inner connection between ideas.

In this confusion of appearances, the tragedy of appreciation reaches its height: those who merely imitate are celebrated, while those who create are misunderstood, resisted, or ignored—until time, distance, and purification finally restore justice to judgment.

The genuinely superior individual may dislike posthumous fame and may suffer from the lack of admiration and recognition during his lifetime; yet, for the progress of society as a whole, the ingratitude of contemporaries is often a blessing. An admired genius inevitably falls—against his own will—under the spell of mass suggestion. In return for admiration, he must endure the puerilities, the bodily and mental deformities, the grotesque beliefs and crude aspirations of the multitude. More than that, he is often compelled to invent flattering theories in their defense and to compromise between his pure, elevated ideals and the coarse, earthbound desires of the masses.

Those who believe that geniuses must be stimulated in their creative work by admiration, social recognition, or material reward do not understand the true nature of genius. They fail to recognize its spontaneous, irresistibly impulsive, and self-rewarding character. They do not see how necessary psychical isolation, social obscurity, or the absence of public prominence is for preserving the height and purity of truly creative work.

The envious man praises one individual only in order to attack another more effectively, or he praises a minor merit so as to gain easier access to the condemnation of what is essential. In such cases, praise becomes a weapon, a tool of concealed hostility, a means of appearing impartial in order to win the confidence of readers or listeners.

Language and thought are always an incomplete and discontinuous translation of conscious mental life; conscious activity itself is discontinuous in relation to the vast realm of subconscious and unconscious processes; and these, in turn, are imperfect translations of the continuous stream of external influences acting upon our senses. Hence arises the great difficulty of grasping the real thoughts of a genius behind his words—especially when he invests old terms with new meanings.

Artistic and technological geniuses embody their creations in tangible, visible, concrete forms. For this reason, they are more likely to be appreciated during their lifetime and within their own nation than thinkers, scientists, or philosophers, whose achievements belong to the invisible but profoundly real world of ideas and moral insight. Moreover, the works of the former often possess immediate, practical utility, whereas scientific and philosophical creations exert their influence indirectly, potentially, or only in the future.

In modern psychology, the obsession with experimentation and calculation has become so widespread and prestigious that it is pursued even where observation alone would yield the same results with far less effort, or where no meaningful results are likely at all. This is a form of scientific idolatry—a fetishism of numbers and apparatus. We forget that experimentation and calculation are merely tools of verification, instruments of the intellect, and that their value depends entirely on the intellectual capital brought to them. Respect for the method is often transferred uncritically to the experimenter, even when he has no clear aim and reaches no significant conclusion, and when the deductions drawn from heaps of figures and pseudo-facts are so trivial that even mockery would be generous.

An intelligence that is easily readable on the face is usually an intelligence confined to the surface. Genuine intellectual activity occurs at deeper levels and does not readily reveal itself outwardly. A lively face may indicate quick perception and practical cleverness, but disinterested intellectual depth is not constantly alert to external events. On the contrary, intense inner mental activity often accompanies a seemingly sleepy expression and moments of perceptual dullness.

Under normal conditions—excluding cases of physiological mimicry, whether the simulation of unfelt emotions or the suppression of genuine inner states—physiognomy reveals less the momentary thoughts or conscious motives of a person than his habitual mental condition, inherited temperament, and unconscious emotional tendencies. It discloses not so much what one is at a given moment, but what one tends to be through heredity—the deeper strata of the soul. The genius has neither the dull, expressionless face of the philistine nor the alert, calculating look of the practical business man. His features reflect calm, serenity, dreaminess, and a dwelling in distant realms of thought, with only partial participation in immediate surroundings.

Our parasite-ridden social organization, with its deceitful and predatory ruling class above and its oppressed, fear-ridden masses below, has produced a striking contradiction between physiognomy and real character or intelligence. Members of the exploiting class often develop such refined powers of mimicry and simulation—an exaggerated cultivation of form and appearance—that deception becomes organic and even anatomically expressed. They possess larger heads, higher foreheads, expressive eyes, confident or defiant postures, and smiling, reassuring faces—appearing more intelligent, kind, or courageous than the intellectual proletarians, beside whom they reveal themselves as intellectual dwarfs and moral cowards. They perfect the outward appearance inherited from their parvenu ancestors, while allowing even the little inner substance that once enabled those ancestors to rise to evaporate. Among the toiling classes, on the other hand—forced to suppress individuality and serve merely as instruments of exploitation—we encounter men whose intelligence has survived persecution by hiding behind insignificant or dull-looking faces; whose courage cannot be guessed from timid features or shrunken bodies; whose kindness and self-sacrificing love of humanity are contradicted by sorrowful or embittered expressions. The marks of oppression, fear, submission, and worry stamped upon their faces reveal their class, but not their true individuality, nor the noble, courageous, and tender hearts concealed within hardened, unattractive exteriors.

Every individual, superior or inferior, must be judged within his own sphere of interests, for interest is the primary condition of attention. What we do not care about, we scarcely notice; what we scarcely notice, we judge poorly or unjustly. A poetic genius may be a weak logician; a profound philosopher may be a superficial scientist—yet he remains no less a profound philosopher.

The true genius must always be, to some degree, a philosopher. Even if not born as one, by advancing far enough within his own field, he inevitably crosses into others and confronts the question of their unity and underlying harmony. In seeking connections between all forms of knowledge, he is led—consciously or unconsciously—into philosophy.

The speculative thinker, the philosopher, is primarily concerned with general, ultimate, and comprehensive views—with higher syntheses of concepts and with complete world-views (Weltanschauungen). For this reason, he cannot expend his energy on observation and experimentation, which by their very nature must restrict themselves to a single aspect of a single class of facts. His position is comparable to that of the workingman in our highly specialized modern industrial organization, who confines his labor to an almost infinitesimal detail, while the manager or financial speculator surveys the entire complex field of an industry—its production, distribution, transportation, sales, consumption, and even the influencing or bribing of government.

Just as, in the industrial world, an intelligent, sober, ambitious, unscrupulous, and hypocritical workingman may rise to the position of foreman in a particular department, then—by analogy—acquire a superficial but practically sufficient knowledge of the other departments, and finally, at a later age, reach the top as manager or active partner; so, in the intellectual world, an observer or experimenter of superior intelligence may advance to the rank of scientist. From his own specialty he may, by analogy, gain a tolerable understanding of allied sciences, and eventually, in maturity, rise to the level of philosophical speculation.

Conversely, just as a man endowed with inborn commercial aptitude and favorable financial circumstances need not begin as a simple specialized laborer, but may from the outset gather information about the whole manufacturing process and its interrelations, so a man with an innate speculative gift and an independent character may assimilate the observations and experiments produced by scientific workers in various related fields. On the basis of this assimilated knowledge—very rarely worked out by him personally—he may then begin to speculate.

As workingmen are content with simple, monotonous, and unrefined food, so the scientific workingman—the pure observer or experimenter, the non-speculative scientist—rests satisfied with primitive intellectual nourishment: raw, isolated, and often uninterpreted observations of a single kind. The intellectual aristocrat, the thinker, on the other hand, requires a broad range of varied and specially prepared intellectual food. He needs observations gathered from many fields, interpreted, analyzed, and synthesized into larger unities. The speculative thinker is endowed by nature with intellectual capital—that is, with an inborn capacity to extract the greatest intellectual value from individual experiences, and with a natural aptitude for forming general views, hypotheses, and comprehensive conceptions. He seldom descends into the low regions of brute facts and insignificant details to verify or modify his hypotheses, or to seek suggestions for new ones. Such detailed verification and correction he usually leaves to scientists, observers, and experimenters who, possessing less or no intellectual capital, limit their activity to elaborating the suggestions of the former and preparing the raw material needed for further intellectual construction.

This is the proper role of the scientist, especially of the pure observer or experimenter, even though such workers often prefer to deny their anonymous intellectual employer or benefactor, and even though they occasionally attempt to emancipate themselves from him.

Reputation and success presuppose ability among other qualities, but the reverse is not necessarily true: ability alone does not lead to reputation. Given favorable circumstances, even a small degree—or merely the appearance—of superiority may suffice to secure public recognition. For this reason, living superior individuals cannot be judged by their reputation. Nor is it justifiable, as Galton suggests, to regard a man as superior merely because he enjoys prominence, influence, or power—because he has the opportunity to make noise, to appropriate and apply the ideas of others, and, in short, to do what almost any average man could do if placed in the same position.

The analytical writer, who moves only in straight lines—who takes up a single thread of thought at a time and follows it step by step—has far greater chances of being widely read, quickly understood, and rapidly rewarded with reputation, wealth, or position than the synthetic writer. The latter, while describing a part, cannot help revealing the whole; while following a definite line of thought A–B–C–D, he feels compelled to indicate, at least in passing, the parallel and collateral lines A'–B'–C'–D', the higher and lower principles connected with them, their relations, their implications, and their possible applications.

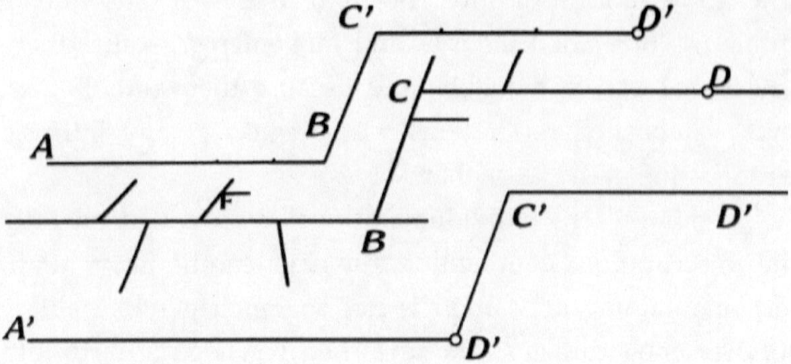

The synthetic thinker therefore produces far fewer books than the analytical thinker, and incomparably fewer than the purely erudite compiler.

In a single work he offers a wealth of new and fertile ideas, each of which an analytical writer could easily stretch into an entire volume by diluting it with superfluous details, illustrations, repetitions, and well-known commonplaces.

To possess abilities is one thing; to know how to convert them into wealth, fame, and success is quite another and constitutes a separate kind of ability; to acquire wealth, fame, and success by exploiting the abilities of others is a third kind of ability—an immoral and parasitic one.

If genius and fame were necessarily linked, we would know the names of the countless anonymous geniuses of the people who condensed their wisdom into proverbs and their noblest sentiments into folk poetry, instead of spreading them out in voluminous printed books.

It is not the genuinely original man—who never rushes to publish ideas the moment they arise, but waits until they have grouped themselves into a harmonious whole, in the manner of a Spinoza—who becomes famous during his lifetime. Fame usually goes to the pseudo- and semi-superior men who inflate their slightest original notion into magazine articles, who know how to exploit topicality, how to fight for and advertise immature, one-sided theories and movements because they are sensational and fashionable, and because their authors already enjoy established reputations, not because of any intrinsic or lasting value in the ideas themselves.

In our present individualistic society, founded on ruthless and unscrupulous competition, the chief condition for attaining and maintaining a position is not so much genuine ability to perform one's duties as the unearned privilege of birth into an influential family, the talent for flattering superiors, the skill of concealing ignorance or incapacity, and the readiness to exploit social inferiors while sharing the spoils with those above.

Only those who naively and hopefully throw themselves wholly into the uncertain struggle of life, without hidden reservations, without the intention of retreating into parasitism or hypocrisy at the first sign of danger or failure, without the readiness to abandon moral principles as soon as they obstruct success—only such people begin early to feel the heavy burden of life's tasks and responsibilities. They are the ones most exposed to paralysis through fear of failure, to premature breakdown, and to being driven by life's obstacles into misery, apathy, mere vegetative existence, or even insanity.

In the so-called sociable man, the critical faculty is overactive and merciless when he judges the disinherited and exploited classes, the newly risen, or superior individuals still unknown to public opinion. The same critical sense, however, falls asleep—or becomes hypocritically indulgent—when he confronts the wealthy, the prominent, or the illustrious. In the first case, he detects banality and defects where there is genuine originality and merit; in the second, his minimizing eye becomes magnifying. The sociable man is superficial in thought, feeling, and action alike. He is friendly with everyone, yet truly a friend of no one. He speaks about everything, but at bottom understands nothing.

Superiority in intelligence can never be tested except through original work. Knowledge may be purely verbal or memorized; reasoning may be nothing more than analogy with problems already solved by others. The mark of real knowledge is the ability to draw new conclusions from it and to apply it independently.

Just as there are "sons of good families" who gain access everywhere without credentials or scrutiny, so there exist words, phrases, and expressions of high repute which, when used by any charlatan in scientific, philosophical, or literary discussion, give him the appearance of a thinker. Our respect for these stereotyped formulas prevents us from examining whether they are legitimate in the context in which they are employed. Thus the superficial humbug hides behind expressions that carry meaning for others but are empty for himself; he exploits symbols of thought just as dishonest politicians exploit symbols of patriotism or morality.

What is true of consecrated expressions holds, though to a lesser degree, for language in general. A thoughtless man can speak without his emptiness being detected, because we naïvely assume that thought always stands behind words.

Just as philistines—and even certain psychologists—fail to understand the psyche of individuals from other classes, nations, or epochs because they mistake superficial differences of language, manners, customs, or dress for essential and inborn distinctions, so the masses, living on very low intellectual levels, fail to grasp the existence of intellectual heights with their wide horizons and pure moral air, where genuine superior men live.

The only "superior" men they recognize and celebrate are the semi- and pseudo-superior ones—those who stand high enough to imitate the loftiness of true superiority, yet remain close enough to the masses to stay within their field of vision, dazzling them with economic success and social prominence rather than with depth, truth, or originality.

Since remunerative occupations and serious life-activities are today very rarely matters of free choice or of specific natural aptitude, a man's character, dominant interests, and real abilities reveal themselves far more clearly in his amusements, in his play, and in those non-lucrative activities in which he freely, gladly, and sincerely takes delight. In play and in reverie, man gives expression to impulses that are partly or wholly suppressed in his bread-winning work. Here he acts without calculation, without the pressure of social expectation or advantage.

Thus, the pseudo-scientist whose investigations are largely plagiarisms and whose scientific activity serves merely as a means of enrichment or vanity will not seek rest or joy in disinterested inquiry, in free discussion, or in thought that lies outside his specialty. He will avoid such pursuits and fill his leisure with anything else, or waste it in idle diversion. The genuine thinker, on the contrary, finds relaxation only in freely chosen intellectual activity: in solitary reflection, in reading, lectures, stimulating conversation, or in walks and travels that unexpectedly supply material for thought. He never finds rest in the philistine's games or in aimless muscular exertion.

The business man who derives neither inner satisfaction nor sufficient profit from his occupation, and who engages in business not merely to live but from greed or rapacity, seeks relaxation in gambling, card-playing, races, ball games, and prize-fights—activities that imitate the competitive excitement and warfare of commercial life. The wage laborer who toils day after day without hope of improvement will, if not yet completely stultified, find pleasure in listening to agitators and pioneers of a better social order; if already dulled, he seeks forgetfulness in sleep, intoxication, narcotics, coarse joking, mutual teasing, betting, or lotteries.

The modern pseudo-ruler, who no longer has occasion to fight or kill men openly and who has no sincere wish to leave the world better than he found it, indulges in boxing, hunting, the killing of animals, or in secret intrigue, vindictiveness, and schemes for self-glorification. Among the great mass of modern women, for whom love is the chief or sole concern of life, the serious-minded and sexually honest—when not actually in love—seek relaxation in novels dealing with love; the sexually dishonest devote their leisure to flirtation and pleasure resorts; the married, sexually honest women of the well-to-do classes find diversion in gossip, endless talk, slander, dilettantism, or private philanthropy. Only the poor workingman's wife, faithful to her domestic duties, scarcely finds any time at all for amusement.

The idler, whose entire existence is consumed by play, luxury, pleasure-seeking, and amorous pursuits, stands even lower than animals, which at least have one serious task in life—the securing of food for themselves and their young. The honest man who barely earns a living for his family seeks no relaxation; and the fortunate individual whose profession coincides with his vocation—the realization of his natural gifts—hardly needs any. He who truly loves his work never seeks pleasure in activities of an opposite nature.

Thus the genuine philanthropist does not delight in the plutocrat's fault-finding with the poor; the true scholar cannot waste time on gossip, platitudes, petty ambition, or athletics; the genuine athlete has a sincere aversion to intellectual pursuits; the disinterested leader of men has no time for idle amusements;

and the genuine labor leader does not feel at ease at the tables or in the salons of exploiters.

Admiration Without Adherence

We may admire a great thinker without accepting his doctrines, once we recognize that the fundamental ideas upon which he builds—consciously or unconsciously—are often imposed upon him through physiological or social heredity. A masterful logical structure may rest upon a shaky or illogical foundation. Hence, the amount of objective truth attained by a genius cannot always serve as the sole measure of his greatness. For those geniuses who are free to choose their foundations, objectivity is the true criterion; for all geniuses alike, inner logic and consistency remain the general standard. The work of genius forms an organic, living whole—an intellectual organism—rather than a neatly systematized arrangement of knowledge. The opposite is true of non-original writers.

The Treatment of Superior Men and their Social Usefulness

In practice, we treat men not according to what they truly are, but according to what they claim to be. The pseudo-superior man instinctively exploits this mixture of politeness, fear, and cowardice in average civilized people. The genuine superior man, absorbed in higher pursuits and restrained by modesty, neither claims nor demands the recognition he deserves. Out of fear, self-interest, or submission, society bows before those who assume authority, affect importance, and shrink from no means—however base—of maintaining it.

The ideal, straight-minded, and poor individual is exposed to having his merits ignored, distorted into defects, or at best undervalued, while his weaknesses are exaggerated or invented.

He lacks the time, patience, and means to proclaim his worth. He cannot compete with pseudo-superior men who loudly and persistently impress their supposed superiority upon the intellectually blind masses, which lack both the will and the capacity to examine the validity of such claims.

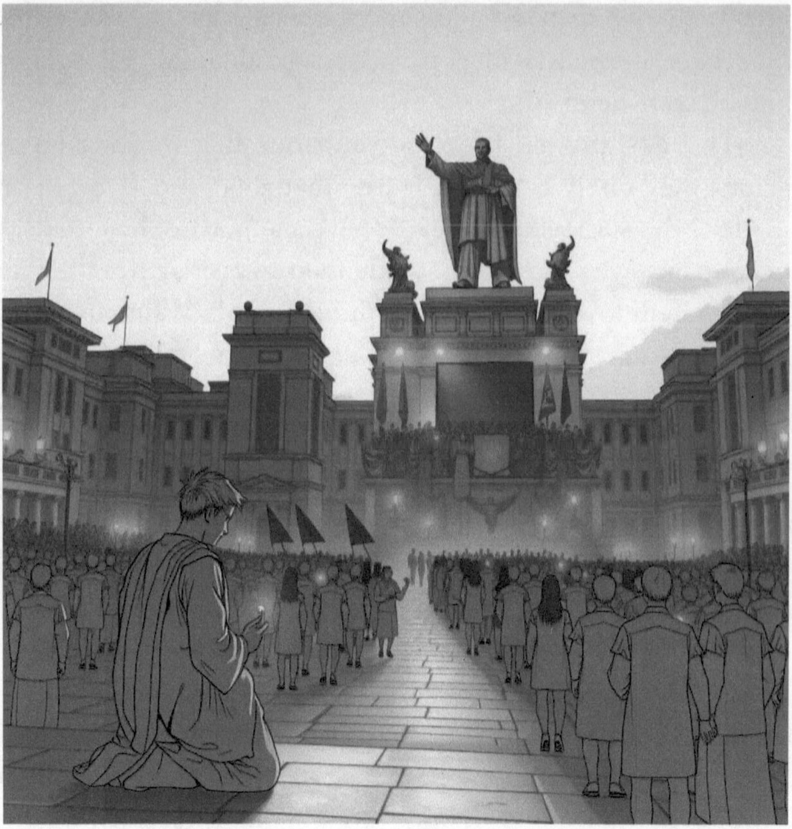

By pseudo-superior, one must not understand a man entirely devoid of merit or usefulness. Superiority cannot be simulated where nothing exists. Simulation consists in exaggerating what is present in small measure; in giving permanence and intentionality to what occurred only occasionally; in presenting egotism and self-pity as altruism and sympathy. The usefulness and harm of pseudo-superior men in the intellectual world correspond to that of middlemen in commerce. They are a necessary evil so long as producers and consumers—geniuses and those thirsting for knowledge—remain widely separated and do not form a single class. Semi-superior men—poets, novelists, emotional writers, many social reformers—are generally more honest and socially more useful intermediaries than pseudo-superior men such as professional preachers, journalists, most professors, academical philosophers, and official scientists.

The most prominent pseudo-superior men are consummate actors; they rarely betray their true thoughts or motives. Yet no matter how successfully they deceive the masses, historians, or even themselves, they cannot hide their hypocrisy from the rare independent lovers of truth who judge them by a simple maxim: Tell me whom you favor, and I shall tell you who you are. If you favor hypocrites, mercenary flatterers, and self-seekers, then you belong to their kind.

The morally pseudo-superior men—professional moralists, preachers, and the majority of leaders and organizers of philanthropic, labor, political, and ethical institutions—present themselves as intermediaries between moral geniuses and the masses. Moral geniuses contribute ethically original ideas, visions for improving the condition of the people, for raising the moral level of society, and for strengthening human solidarity. They do so without expecting, and without receiving, any reward beyond inner moral satisfaction. The financial and exploiting classes, on the other hand, provide the material means necessary for maintaining such institutions, but only on the condition that the pseudo-superior intermediaries do not interfere with, expose, or challenge the criminal and parasitical methods of the exploiters.

The moral genius is too honest and too disinterested to accept support under such conditions. At the same time, he is too poor, too isolated, and too unsupported to carry on the moral struggle entirely on his own. Moral progress is therefore left largely in the hands of pseudo-superior men who are willing to compromise between their professed convictions and their personal interests—men who are prepared to serve the people only insofar as doing so also serves themselves. From such semi-mercenary guardians of morality, no radical, swift, or genuine cure of social evils can reasonably be expected.

The pseudo-superior man is not a promoter but rather an obstacle to truth, morality, art, progress, and social happiness. He turns everything into a profession, a business, a source of income and prestige. He embraces a new truth, idea, sentiment, or ethical, religious, or social movement only so long as it can be made profitable to himself. Yet he lives just as comfortably on the fears, prejudices, ignorance, superstitions, and conflicts of the masses as he does on the higher aspirations, ideals, and creative achievements of superior men. Like the middleman in economic life, he has no genuine interest in either side: neither in producers nor consumers, neither in employers nor employees, neither in rulers nor ruled. He exploits both, keeps them apart while pretending to reconcile them, and often inflames antagonisms under the guise of healing them.

He has no interest in the disappearance of social evils or in the triumph of the good, for such outcomes would mark the end of his profitable and illustrious parasitic career. His thirst for authority is merely rapacity in a softened and disguised form. Pseudo-superior men are the merchants of the intellectual world: they commercialize, capitalize, sell, and often claim credit for ethical, religious, scientific, and philosophical ideas that they have appropriated from genuine intellectual producers. In this respect, they are even more unscrupulous than material dealers, who are at least sometimes compelled to acknowledge and compensate those they exploit. While pretending to advance human progress, the pseudo-superior man in reality obstructs it.

Those who lack any genuine capacity to create, invent, compose, think, or lead often constitute themselves critics, advisers, and teachers, arrogantly prescribing methods of action, standards of thought, rules of language, and laws for both the masses and the geniuses. Those who habitually evade or violate laws frequently transform themselves into legislators and guardians of legality. They devise legal, financial, and institutional mechanisms to bind both superior men and the masses, capturing the fruits of collective labor for themselves. Institutions originally intended to serve the public good are converted into instruments of exploitation, domination, and intellectual stagnation.

At times, however, these pseudo-superior men become entangled in the very legal fictions and hollow idealistic rhetoric they have created, and are forced to remain trapped until an escape is found. Meanwhile, genuinely ideal individuals and the masses slowly reclaim portions of their lost freedom. Modern economic, political, educational, and social systems have grown so complex, interconnected, and international that they increasingly threaten to escape the coordinated control of pseudo-superior men, and thus hold the promise of being reclaimed by society at large—by the honest and intelligent elements of humanity.

Under the present reign of hypocrisy fostered by competitive struggle, there is no danger in speaking of idealism, for everyone does so, even the crudest materialist. The superior man becomes an object of hostility only when he dares to act in accordance with his ideals, when he naïvely assumes that those who speak the language of idealism mean it in practice. In reality, the principles they proclaim are not meant for daily use. When the ideal man fails, he stands alone; when he succeeds, the entire world rallies around him, and pseudo-idealists hasten to claim him as their leader and inspiration. The ideal man is an enfant terrible to his acquaintances. Privately they may admire him, but publicly they avoid him, for in public life they wear the same masks as everyone else. He is deeply disillusioned if he mistakes private friendliness for public loyalty.

The destiny of the ideal superior man has always been, and will always remain, one of solitude and renunciation. Socrates, despised by the sophists of his time and condemned by the ruling pseudo- and semi-superior men, would fare no better today were he to return. Those who now quote and glorify him would be embarrassed to associate with him. Likewise, those who preach in the name of Jesus would likely shun him as an inconvenient, unadaptable revolutionary, and might even exclude him from the very church that claims his name.

Mutual Misunderstanding Between Superior and Average Man

Genuine superior men are often ridiculed—if not openly, then covertly—by average and pseudo-superior men for their simplicity, modesty, and belief in immortality and enduring values. In turn, the superior man pities the average and pseudo-superior men for their fleeting ambitions and perishable pleasures. In truth, the two groups misunderstand each other. Both act logically within the limits of their nature. What is illusory or unattainable for one class may be real and sufficient for the other. One who expects everything from immediate society cannot act like one who works for humanity across generations.

The clear-minded, truth-loving, altruistic superior man feels boredom—but not personal offense—when confronted with the writings of obscure, mystical, self-worshiping pseudo-superior men. They, however, feel personally attacked and irritated by the impersonal clarity and sincerity of his work, for it exposes, without naming them, the emptiness of their pretensions. Every individual, in judging others, inevitably takes himself—or at best his own aspirations—as a standard of measurement. The matter-of-fact, truth-loving, clear-headed person cannot help being somewhat prejudiced against the formal, insincere, vainglorious, self-glorifying, or mystical type. His instinctive contempt for untruthfulness and obscurity leads him to underestimate the small measure of genuine talent or goodness that may nevertheless exist in such men. Yet even more unjust is the attitude of the self-seeker, the insincere, the mystical type toward the truth-loving individual. He appreciates superior skill or talent only in members of his own class, and only so long as such appreciation does not endanger his own glory or interests.

Every man admires—and at the same time betrays—himself in others. He admires in them what corresponds to his own attainments and aspirations. The insincere, together with the masses of blind imitators, display verbal, outward, and interested admiration for any type of man whom fortune has crowned with success and popularity. Hence, when we lack the possibility of judging men by our own direct insight, it is not enough to collect opinions indiscriminately. We must attach the greatest weight to the judgments of truth-loving colleagues whose interests are neither opposed to nor entangled with those of the person under evaluation. More value must be given to inner, spontaneous, unconsciously revealed admiration than to outward, calculated, deliberately expressed praise. It matters less what verdict is pronounced than who pronounces it, and why.

A genius is very rarely a good critic. He finds expression too easily for thoughts and feelings that others struggle to articulate; he discovers answers to questions that others ask in vain. For this reason, he cannot easily appreciate the difficulty, the inaccessibility, or even the value of his own findings for ordinary minds. His own methods are too personal, too irrepressible, to allow him to judge fairly the paths chosen by other geniuses. Measuring others by himself, he often fails to recognize the importance of mere talent for the great mass. Standing too high above it, he cannot properly estimate distances in lower regions; he scarcely perceives the difference between philistines and talented men, or between varying degrees of talent. Yet he is better equipped to appreciate geniuses greater than himself, or those who stand immediately below him, provided they belong to his own or a related domain. He lacks real understanding, however, for geniuses of an entirely different type.

The born critic occupies an intermediate position—above the average mind, below genius. From this vantage point, he is better able to estimate talent and differences in talent, though less capable of judging differences among geniuses. A man of genius may nevertheless be a sound critic in fields where he possesses taste or talent but no originality.

We can judge accurately only what is not too far above or below us. Thus, the semi-scientific observer or experimenter who mocks speculative thinkers and generalizations in fields unknown to him may feel pride when he himself arrives at a general view within his own specialty, because there he can appreciate the guiding power of speculation. Similarly, in industrial life, the ordinary worker may understand the necessity of a foreman yet fail to grasp the importance of an engineer or superintendent.

When the self-conceited find fault with everyone who does not bow before them, it is because they seek to highlight their imagined greatness. By belittling others, they attempt to magnify themselves and derive pleasure from stripping others of their hard-won reputation. They spare only those willing to pay tribute and become their intellectual dependents.

When the genuinely superior man discovers faults, limitations, or pettiness, it is not because he is blind to merit or greatness, nor because he delights in depreciation. Were that the case, he would spare his admirers and enjoy his own uniqueness. In truth, he cannot avoid perceiving smallness when he measures others by the standards of his own achievements and aspirations.

Pseudo-superior men show remarkable ingenuity in diminishing the genuine qualities of genius. Philosophical depth that penetrates beneath superficial historical change to enduring realities is labeled a lack of historical sense. The refusal to participate in frivolous amusements is branded as absence of humor. The moral genius is accused of impracticality, inadaptability, or anarchistic tendencies when he condemns a competitive, laissez-faire system that rewards greed, vanity, and one-sided degeneration. Mental richness and versatility are dismissed as lack of concentration; frankness and open-heartedness are ridiculed as naïveté; preserved idealism is called childishness or foolishness.

Cosmopolitanism—the refusal to revere artificial, transient national or racial distinctions—has not yet been baptized as a lack of geographical sense, though it might well be. The subordination of immediate material interests to truth and enduring spiritual aims is interpreted as unfitness or lack of business ability, as if unfitness for evil were blameworthy, as if one deficiency could explain a surplus of ability elsewhere, or as if striving upward could be explained by an inability to remain below. In reality, it demands far greater intelligence, courage, foresight, and a higher form of adaptability to live by honest, socially useful work than by parasitic or deceptive methods; to pursue lasting, universal goods rather than fleeting personal gains; to renounce petty ambitions rather than cling to them; to confront exploiters and pseudo-rulers rather than flatter them; to enlighten the masses instead of exploiting their ignorance; to express new, bold ideas in plain language rather than disguise stale views in obscure phrases. It is not hatred of a parasitic minority but love for the honest masses that drives the moral genius—whether socialist, anarchist, or communist—to oppose the rule of the so-called upper class. He is accused of fomenting class hatred, because this sounds more acceptable than the truth: resistance to exploitation. Rarely is he credited with dissolving the more dangerous hatreds between races, nations, sects, and parties that parasitic minorities cultivate for their own benefit.

Self-Appreciation

Beyond the confusion between sentiment and reason, and between the desire for superiority and belief in one's superiority, there exists another reason why women are often more self-conceited than men, the rich more than the poor, children more than adults, and socially prominent pseudo-superior men more than obscure genuine ones. They are seldom contradicted, especially in opinions about themselves, and are continually surrounded by favor-seekers and flatterers. Continuous unchallenged admiration gradually hardens illusion into conviction, and self-deception becomes self-certainty.

The pseudo-superior man is complacently absorbed in what he knows—or believes he knows—and in his imagined superiority over the masses. The genuine superior man, by contrast, is preoccupied with what he does not yet know, with what he longs to understand, and with his own distance from the ideals he pursues. The aristocratic philistine's, and the pseudo-superior man's, idealization of themselves and of the existing order is a clear sign of their lack of progressiveness and of their merely illusory originality. It also betrays a dim awareness of their own deficiencies, of their inability to improve themselves, to examine themselves fearlessly, to transform their environment, or to satisfy in any genuine way the inborn human impulse to strive upward.

Great minds usually release into the intellectual world ideas whose range they themselves cannot fully foresee. They form concepts, laws, and comprehensive views without knowing the countless particular cases that will later be brought under them, or the vast sphere of their applicability. The disciples of such men are often naïve enough to assume that the master must also perceive and draw every possible conclusion from his own ideas. They are therefore deeply disappointed when they discover in their teacher the same blindness as in ordinary men with regard to certain applications of his own theories—applications that seem obvious and self-evident to the disciples.

The superior man often becomes capable of judging his own creations only after a lapse of time, and especially after producing better ones. He then views earlier works in the light of later achievements, forgetting how much labor and suffering the former once cost him, and thus gaining a more objective perspective. For the genius, personal attachment to his creations is proportionate to the effort and pain expended on them.

The sub-conscious and un-conscious, which appear so mysterious to the psychologist and the thinker whose mental life has reached a high degree of clarity, are in reality no more enigmatic than consciousness itself. Indeed, they may be considered less problematic, for they represent the raw material, the cradle and the grave of all thought, just as chaos and disorder in the outer world give rise to, and later threaten to engulf, order and cosmos. Consciousness, clarity, harmony, and purposeful activity emerge from disorder and remain perpetually exposed to relapse into vagueness, disconnection, and unconsciousness.

All original thought is spontaneous and involuntary: it rises from the sub-conscious into the light of awareness, overcoming resistance and repression caused by the pain of dislocating established systems of feeling and belief. Like many women in childbirth, original thinkers often dislike their new ideas while they are still forming, and even immediately after their birth.

Their affection for these spiritual children grows with the effort made to defend, develop, and perfect them.

Only the superior man endowed with objective self-introspection can truly appreciate himself. The average man measures his own worth by the esteem granted him by his surroundings. His resentment of criticism and hostility toward critical minds betray an obscure awareness of his lack of solid merit. The pseudo-superior man's hunger for popularity, honors, titles, and high positions, and his eagerness to be credited with qualities he scarcely possesses, spring not only from a desire to deceive others but also from a need to deceive himself. His ambition far outstrips his real powers. He believes in his own importance only in proportion to the admiration he manages to elicit. Lacking confidence in his true abilities, he requires constant external persuasion and collective hypnosis to sustain belief in his greatness. Dissatisfied with his real self, he seeks consolation in a self-image maintained by auto- and hetero-suggestion.

Criteria of Genius

Different kinds of genius are practically incommensurable. Each must be judged by a distinct qualitative and quantitative standard. Emotional genius is measured by beauty, observational genius by objectivity or fidelity to reality, theoretical genius by truth and logical consistency, technical genius by utility, and moral genius by the degree of social happiness it promotes.

This does not mean that a work of art, for example, should be judged solely by beauty and without regard to truth or morality. It means only that beauty is its primary criterion, while truth, utility, and moral significance function as secondary qualities. A genuine work of art contains a maximum of beauty and an optimum—not an excess—of these secondary ends. If two works are equally beautiful, then secondary criteria decide which embodies greater genius.

Seen in this light, both doctrines—art for art's sake and art as necessarily moral—appear equally one-sided and immature. A novel or artwork need not have an explicit moral purpose. If, however, it implicitly conveys truth or ethical insight, its value is enhanced. When moral teaching becomes too explicit, art degenerates into didacticism.

The distaste many feel for so-called "novels with a purpose" arises not because art and ethics are incompatible, but either because the work is artificial and intellectually dishonest—pretending to extract a moral from events when the lesson was inserted in advance—or because its readers belong to classes for whom ethics is unwelcome in any form. We judge men and works by the claims they make. A work that adopts an artistic form while serving primarily moral aims may be undervalued if it fails to justify its aesthetic pretensions. Many themes would be better appreciated if expressed plainly in prose rather than clothed in verse.

In general, we overestimate intelligence where we expect little of it, and underestimate it where we expect much. Thus animal flashes of intelligence surprise us because animals make no claim to intellect, while the limited intelligence of human imbeciles passes unnoticed because men pride themselves on their cleverness. Similarly, works are judged not only by what they are, but by what they promise to be.

In all these domains, the decisive distinction remains the same: the pseudo-superior man clings to appearances, self-satisfaction, and external validation; the genuine superior man is driven by inner striving, dissatisfaction with himself, and fidelity to ideals that lie beyond his present reach.

Although the criteria of genius are still largely qualitative, subjective, and seemingly arbitrary, they are nevertheless applied—silently, implicitly, and often unconsciously. It is difficult, for example, to decide between two purely lyrical poets who both give equally adequate expression to the same human passions. Yet if one of them is capable of interweaving philosophical reflection—if, alongside beauty, he implicitly offers a certain measure of insight or truth—we instinctively judge him the greater poet, even when his emotional expression is no richer than that of the other. Of two purely scientific or philosophical thinkers, the greater is the one whose generalizations are wider, whose thought embraces a larger field of phenomena. And of two thinkers whose conceptions are equally broad, the greater is the one who is more many-sided—who, in addition to truth, also conveys poetry, usefulness, and moral insight.

Appreciation and Reward of Genius under the Capitalist Regime

Just as, in our chaotic and predatory economic world, workers and producers are insufficiently organized to choose their own supervisors, leaders, or rulers from among the most broad-minded, many-sided, and humane within their own ranks—and are therefore compelled to submit either to self-appointed slave-drivers incapable of production, or to superiors imposed by parasitic rulers and exploiters—so, too, in the intellectual world, genuine poets, artists, dramatists, scientists, philosophers, inventors, and creative thinkers are too poor, too scattered, and too isolated to elect their own critics from among the most comprehensive and discerning minds of their own class. They are thus forced to bow before self-anointed, power- or fame-seeking pseudo-critics, or before professional, capital-employed censors—publishers, editors, reviewers, official educators and preachers—who, being themselves aborted thinkers, mentally sterile and incapable of original creation, often lacking even taste or unbiased judgment, monopolize the channels of publicity.

These monopolizers arrogate to themselves the right to dictate what shall be written or spoken and in what manner; the right to sit in judgment on the creations of others; the right to distribute praise and honor among their dependents; the right to grant or withhold publicity at will; the right to claim undeserved credit for having "discovered" or "encouraged" certain geniuses who would have risen regardless, because their genre happened to be fashionable; and the right to escape blame for having discouraged, corrupted, ruined, or driven into prostitution countless other geniuses who were merely ahead of their time—or, more accurately, not acceptable to the exploiting interests.

So long as intellectual producers depend for recognition on such pseudo-critics or disguised censors, and for their livelihood on the sale of their works to the idle rich—whose superficial, fickle, and capricious tastes must first be flattered—so long as the means of economic production and distribution, and the intellectual channels of information and publicity (including those that call themselves socialistic), remain monopolized by small cliques and parasitic minorities that more often cooperate than compete, this state of affairs must continue. Under such conditions, access to the press, the pulpit, the platform, and academic positions is granted chiefly to pliable, confused, and pervertible writers who are willing to serve the interests of capitalist exploiters; who submit to the judgment of incompetent usurpers of authority; who suppress or distort truth on command; who intoxicate the people with empty wit and sensational excitement; who hypnotize the masses into worshiping false heroes and pursuing spurious aims.

Meanwhile, the honest, clear-headed intellectual producers who stand for truth, enlightenment, emancipation, and the uplift of humanity—and who care little for honors conferred by incompetent authorities—are relentlessly pushed into obscurity, ridicule, poverty, despair, and stripped of everything except the faint hope of posthumous recognition. Under a regime where the channels of publicity are owned by capital and controlled by pseudo-critics, genuine original thinkers rarely succeed.

They spend their best years producing work worthy of attention and gratitude, only to find that recognition and material reward go instead to unscrupulous phrase-mongers who first secure control over publicity or popularity, and then sell—often at high prices—the intellectual products they have stolen or cheaply acquired from poor, unknown, and unobtrusive original minds.

This mirrors the economic world, where the indispensable labor of farmers and industrial workers is poorly rewarded or ignored, while the sham services of financial speculators are richly compensated.

These speculators first present themselves as useful intermediaries between producers and consumers, and then deliberately drive the two further apart in order to exact tribute from both. Likewise, many college professors and official scientists who own or edit scholarly journals do not genuinely aim to disseminate knowledge, despite their claims. Their hidden purpose, beyond financial gain, is to levy toll on poor, original students and independent thinkers by barring them from access to readers, much as medieval robber barons intercepted merchants on the road to market. Another aim of these intellectual monopolists is mutual glorification and self-immortalization within closed circles, along with the extraction of undeserved recognition from writers in other regions or countries, traded in exchange for reciprocal praise in their own publications.

Thus, under a system where intellectual life is filtered through capital and controlled by parasitic intermediaries, genius is neither fairly judged nor justly rewarded; it is tolerated only when it can be exploited, and suppressed whenever it threatens to illuminate, liberate, or transform.

End of the Chapter

Chapter-9.
Vital Ideals and the Psychology of Genius:
Health, Decline, and Creation

This chapter probes the fragile frontier where genius, health, and decline intersect. It challenges myths that link creativity with madness, distinguishes progressive from regressive originality, and reveals how vital energy, adaptation, and mental equilibrium shape true creation—offering a framework for recognizing fertile genius and resisting seductive but destructive illusions.

Normal and Abnormal Ideals

A healthy, vigorous mind turns its gaze toward the future and seeks there the realization of its ideals. A diseased, exhausted, senile, or declining mind, by contrast, idealizes the past. What is true of the individual holds equally true of entire epochs and literary or intellectual schools. There are ages of hope, marked by a surplus of vital energy, and ages of depression and despair, marked by a deficit of life force.

The ideals of morbid, exhausted, decadent, weak, despairing, insane, impotent, or unproductive individuals lie behind them, in the past, in the realm of sterile dreams, and spring from a longing for external help. These ideals express themselves in romanticism; in vague, idealistic, or nebulous philosophy; in mysticism; in the aspiration toward Nirvana; in ancestor-worship; in animal worship or totemism; in servile hero-worship; in magic; in belief in miracles and messianic deliverance; in fatalism and dogmatism; in the worship of gods; in paternalistic and hierarchical government; in blind reverence for official or institutional wisdom; in obedience to conventions, traditions, precedents, and stereotyped ways of acting; in submission to fashion; in pleasure-seeking; in slave-hunting, warfare, militarism, parasitism, and deception.

The ideals of vigorous, healthy, hopeful, progressive, sane, productive, self-reliant, and resourceful individuals, on the other hand, lie ahead of them, in the future, in the realm of possibilities. They spring from a desire for purposeful activity and self-realization. These ideals find expression in realism; in fearless confrontation with facts; in scientific research; in clear thinking; in free and courageous thought; in belief in causation and economic determinism; in the reverence for humanity; in democracy; in the popularization of knowledge; in socialism, communism, anarchism, cooperation, fairness, sincerity, and respect for logic and reason. Ancestor-worship, the idealization of the "fathers," and the cult of the dead are inseparably linked with blind submission to existing powers and self-appointed rulers. Those in authority promote unquestioning reverence for the past, just as they support other stultifying cults, in order to secure their own posthumous glory and to prevent even future generations from critically examining their motives and actions.

Sane and Insane Genius

The creative act of genius is the intellectual counterpart of childbirth and is preceded by a period of intellectual pregnancy. Bodily pregnancy and childbirth disturb the organism and may sometimes affect the brain and mind. In the same way, the incubation and elaboration of original ideas can disturb the brain and the psyche, and may even give rise to bodily disorders

When body and mind are hereditarily weak or degenerate, such disturbances do not remain limited to transient discomfort, minor confusion, or fleeting illusions. They may take the form of persistent disorders: chronic disease, mental aberration, delusions, uncontrollable hallucinations, insanity, and in extreme cases, death.

To claim, however, as the famous and influential Lombroso did, that degeneration and insanity are causes or conditions of genius and creativity is as erroneous as claiming that puerperal fever or childbirth-related illness is the cause of childbirth itself. Such ailments may accompany the process, but they neither create nor explain it.

When Lombroso, in reply to his critics, pointed to cases of geniuses who were mentally unstable before producing any work, this can be understood as the result of early intellectual pregnancy combined with inherited psychological fragility—an insufficient resistance to the strain imposed by original thought. Mental instability in such cases is not the source of genius, but the consequence of an organism unable to withstand the tension generated by creative incubation.

If, in some distant future, science were able to prevent the conception of original ideas—especially multiple or excessive conceptions—in genetically fragile individuals, by shielding them from overwhelming environments or from too intense contact with nature and fertilizing ideas, such individuals might be protected from insanity and premature death. Just as conception and pregnancy can be prevented in women, so might excessive intellectual conception one day be regulated.

In the early history of humanity, it is plausible that many women could not endure the strain of childbirth and died after the birth of a first child or became sterile through miscarriage, until the species gradually developed greater resistance and fecundity. A similar process seems to apply to intellectual creation. Many individuals become mentally unbalanced during the incubation or after the birth of original ideas, or become sterile after a first creative act, thereafter contenting themselves with adopting, imitating, or appropriating the intellectual offspring of others.

Few, even now, are the genuinely sane geniuses who remain fertile throughout life—capable of resisting the mental strain inherent in creation and of overcoming the discomfort it entails. Few are those who can resist the temptation to conceive ideas so vast and complex that they stretch the mind beyond its capacity for recovery and stable equilibrium. Many generations will still pass before the majority of human beings become intellectually fertile—before sane genius, in one form or another, becomes the common condition rather than the rare exception.

The philistine is mentally sterile and unproductive.

Most pseudo-superior men—the graphomaniacs, the pseudo-active, the nebulous and mystical writers, the verbose authors, and the loquacious talkers—are not fertile minds but abnormally creative or aborted thinkers. They give birth to shapeless, amorphous, non-viable ideas: fragmentary, premature, monstrous, impracticable mock-conceptions. Aware, however dimly, of their inability to offer quality, completeness, originality, or results, they compensate by drawing attention to quantity—mock prolificness, incessant effort, volume, and noise. Instead of patiently producing and nurturing a limited number of clear, practicable, and harmoniously developing ideas, they pour forth innumerable aborted fragments and pseudo-generalizations which, though seemingly different, are in truth repeated failures to grasp and express the same few thoughts that forever escape them.

What drives these immature minds into morbid, incessant, aimless activity—into abortion and premature expulsion of intellectual embryos, into the thrusting of sham ideas upon an unwilling public—is their dread of the solitary, inward life of meditation required by genuine growth; their inability to endure the inner disturbances, dislocations, and readjustments caused by the expansion of new ideas; their fear of mental breakdown under the strain of intellectual pregnancy; and, not least, their vanity and morbid craving for recognition, their impatience to parade originality before it has matured. Those unfortunate minds that come into contact with such stillborn, miscarried, pestiferous pseudo-ideas are often poisoned intellectually for life. Leisure is not the decisive condition for the manifestation of genius or originality. Psychical isolation and independence are far more important. Indeed, geniuses arise as rarely among idle social classes as among paupers. In villages and small, compact communities—where every individual is known, watched, and judged by all others—a sane person cannot safely display peculiarities without attracting hostility, ostracism, and threats to livelihood. He cannot openly differ, cannot refuse participation in common beliefs and practices, however absurd they may appear to him. In such undifferentiated communities, economic dependence goes hand in hand with intellectual stagnation, for public opinion reigns despotically. There, the only conspicuously original individuals are the insane or semi-insane, whose impulsiveness blinds them to the danger of being different.

With the growth of cities, the division of labor, and anonymous forms of livelihood, society splits horizontally and vertically into classes and sub-classes. One and the same individual may belong economically to one group, intellectually to another, emotionally to a third—or to none at all. Psychical isolation increases; freedom of thought expands. Sane geniuses find opportunities to express ideas and pursue ideals, even if not within the economic class on which they depend. Thus, in a more differentiated and tolerant civilization, genius and insanity gradually diverge. The few cases cited of animals showing both nervosity and unusual ability suggest that physiological factors may sometimes outweigh social ones, but they do not invalidate the general tendency.

The mental horizon of the sane genius resembles a clear sky, illuminated by steady sunlight. That of the insane genius resembles a clouded sky, torn intermittently by dazzling flashes of lightning, preceded and followed by gloom. In the sane genius there is continuity and connection between successive acquisitions; he does not fall from heights already reached. The insane genius, by contrast, is often inferior to his own creations and becomes estranged from his own spiritual offspring.

Both the sane genius and the misanthropic genius behave timidly and awkwardly in philistine society. The difference lies in degree and motive. The sane genius withdraws when excessive self-denial is demanded of him; the misanthropic genius recoils even when no sacrifice is required and economic independence is assured.

The average man is suggestible, subjective, and credulous; the superior man is objective-minded. In the insane genius, auto-suggestibility is tyrannical, anarchic, and fixed-idea driven. The sane genius, by contrast, is internally democratic, consistent, and mentally harmonious.

A sane speculative thinker completes a circuit: his thought begins with facts and reality and, sooner or later, returns to them. Abnormal philosophical speculation starts from a fragment of reality and then short-circuits itself, dissolving into an ocean of pure ideas without ever returning to the solid ground from which it arose. Many so-called idealistic philosophers are either impostors or, if sincere, theoretically insane though not practically so. A sane person may advocate an insane theory; an insane person may proclaim a sane one. What distinguishes sanity from insanity is not merely the quality of ideas, but their quantity, persistence, and motor energy—the degree to which they dominate conduct.

The insane genius pays for superiority with disproportion and disharmony. He gains in one direction what he loses in others; his progress is compensatory. The sane genius—or the great talent—progresses by addition. He may, however, pay for intellectual growth with bodily regression or early stagnation, through an overdevelopment of the head at the expense of the rest of the organism. The normal superior man differs from the average man chiefly in degree; the abnormal differs in kind.

Normality, Abnormality, and Adaptation

The enumeration of many traits of genius throughout this mosaic-like, semi-aphoristic, and therefore seemingly incoherent exposition does not imply that every genius possesses all these qualities at all times or in every field. It means only that a genius may display all of them at certain moments—moments of inspiration—and some of them habitually. It means that such traits may appear occasionally in comprehensive surveys of human knowledge and more frequently within limited domains. The genius possesses more of these qualities than the merely talented individual, and the balanced genius possesses them more steadily and with fewer deficiencies than the unbalanced one.

He who rises to the highest summits of comprehension and human sympathy is more exposed to falling into delusion than the average mind, which rarely ventures beyond the safe plateau of inertia and indifference. Abnormalities and inconsistencies that would be alarming in an average person are not surprising in nascent, inexperienced, exhausted, or declining geniuses. What is truly astonishing is that sane men of talent mistake the vagaries of tired or broken-down geniuses for precious revelations and bestow uncritical veneration upon nonsense, moral lapses, and incoherent advice simply because they proceed from a renowned source.

The fact that many geniuses exhibit nervous instability or mental disequilibrium in childhood does not support the doctrine that genius is a product of degeneration. Genius is creative continuously and is therefore continually exposed to exhaustion. In childhood, its creative force is less visible because it is engaged in reconstructing, rediscovering, and assimilating the intellectual acquisitions of humanity, which later serve as the foundation for original construction. At that stage, the divergence between the genius and ordinary minds is too slight or too suppressed to be readily observed. Potentially, however, the difference is as profound at the beginning as it will ever be in later life.

There is greater permanence, stability, and continuity in our tendencies and abilities than in our concrete activities and achievements; more permanence in the direction of our tendencies than in their particular applications or momentary intensity. There is more continuity of selfhood in our activity taken as a whole than in isolated acts; more in the cooperation of our abilities than in their scattered exercise; more in our physiological, emotional, inherited, and sub-conscious personality than in our psychical, intellectual, acquired, and conscious personality.

There is more permanence in our imitative and practical life than in our creative and theoretical life; more harmony and non-contradiction of selfhood, in essential and vital questions, in a normal individual than in an abnormal one; more in ideals, aims, and methods than in concrete means and subject-matter; more in the mature than in the immature; more equilibrium in many-sided scientific and philosophical geniuses than in one-sided artistic or technological talents; more in truth-, essence-, and thought-seeking minds than in beauty-, form-, or phrase-seeking authors. To declare, as Lombroso did, that genius—whether many-sided or one-sided—is itself an abnormality, a morbid deviation, an intellectual monstrosity, is to assume that the human species is a finished, static product of nature. It is to assume that stagnation and inertia represent mankind's normal state, and that progress is merely an anomaly produced by disturbance, persecution, or agitation. Those, however, who hold that humanity is still growing intellectually and morally—if no longer bodily—and that its apparent stagnation is due to parasitism, oppression, and intra-social criminality, do not seek the norm of intellectual or moral health in the average man. They look instead to the fortunate few: the many-sided and moral geniuses who renounce the pursuit of material success and the favor of parasites in order to escape the enslavement that would stifle the free, harmonious, and socially useful development of their inner life.

To determine the intellectual and moral norm of humanity by taking the average condition of the oppressed masses—who under present conditions can never reach maturity—is as erroneous as calculating the average stature of a race without excluding children and individuals with arrested development. A growing being cannot be measured by averaging its undeveloped specimens. Since we cannot compute the norm of a living, evolving species by statistical means alone, the only rational method is to look toward the most fully developed specimens—toward the many-sided and moral geniuses who have escaped the thwarting influences of an anarchical, competitive, predatory order.

The consistent evolutionist therefore reverses Lombroso's criterion. He re-enthrones the genius—not in the naïve form of blind hero-worship, but in a purified, critical sense. He does not take the modern average man as the standard; rather, he regards the absence of higher, many-sided life-interests as a sign of arrested or thwarted development. He knows that under a future orderly, cooperative, and solidary social organization, the types of men that today form the rule will become the exception. Mental superiority is now rare because it grows upward toward truth and love, and is crushed by caste, convention, petty-mindedness, and parasitic institutions. Philistinism, which never grows beyond those barriers, escapes such repression. Our predatory social organization, which tolerates men chiefly as one-sided tools, is largely responsible for the present divorce between bodily and mental growth, between moral and intellectual development, and even between different intellectual faculties. It produces a majority of mentally stunted philistines and a minority of one-sidedly developed geniuses.

Normal and Abnormal Originality

The violation of social prejudices, customs, and traditions may signify either progressive or regressive originality. It is progressive when such conventions have become meaningless, oppressive, or dangerous. It is regressive—though it may incidentally benefit society—when it springs from inadaptability, impulsiveness, vanity, or the hysterical desire for attention. Progressive originality is calm, patient, persuasive, and unobtrusive; regressive originality is noisy, hasty, harsh, provocative, and self-advertising.

Normal and progressive emotional discontent does not expend itself on trivial, harmless, or blameless persons or institutions, nor does it express itself in petty, envious, or malicious criticism. Normal and progressive intellectual originality does not waste itself on verbal subtleties, insoluble dialectical games, or barren problems. Normal and progressive volitional originality does not chase impracticable, irrational, or merely spectacular schemes, nor does it delight in incessant change for its own sake.

Morbid artistic originality—whether labeled impressionism, luminism, pointillism, futurism, cubism, or by any other name—divorces form from content, magnifies trivial details at the expense of the whole, mistakes eccentricity for creativity, and seeks notoriety through shock. It sacrifices substance to appearance or appearance to substance, lacks both patient observation and creative imagination, and mirrors in the aesthetic realm the parasitic, appearance-hunting tendencies of commercial capitalism.

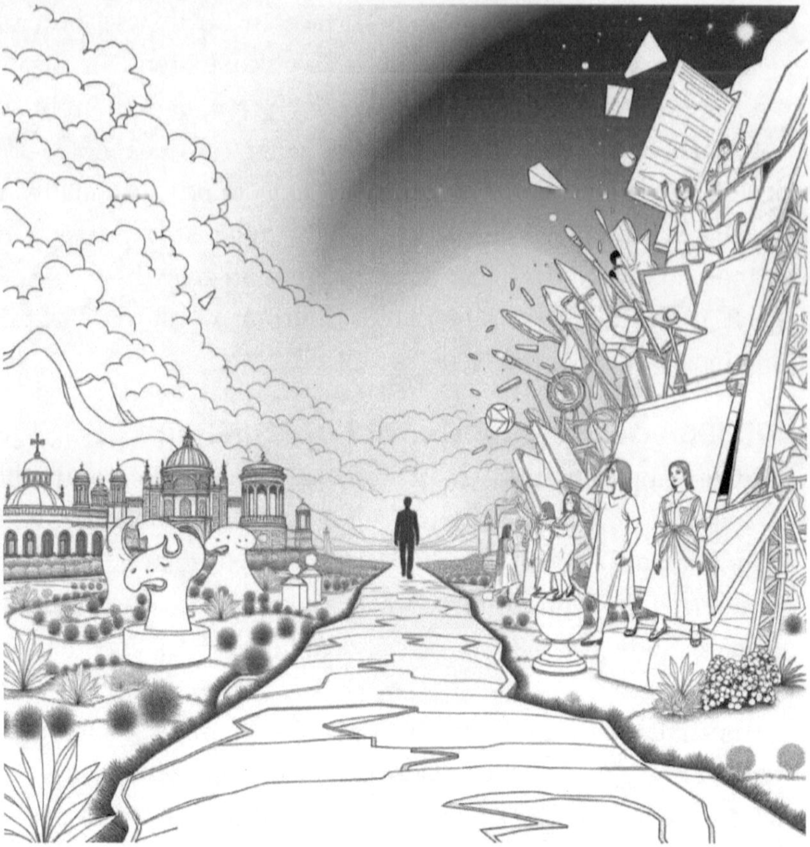

Man is distinguished among animals by his ability to adapt his environment to himself—to create conditions suited to his nature rather than merely submitting to existing ones. This creative adaptability is expressed in industry and social reform. Just as bodily health is not measured by mere conformity to the physical environment, mental sanity cannot be measured by complete conformity to prevailing social norms. There exists a progressive non-conformity as well as a regressive one; therefore, social adaptation alone is an insufficient test of sanity.

In periods of social disorganization, when authority slumbers, obscure personalities often rise suddenly to prominence. Similarly, in disturbed mental states, when higher regulatory centers are inactive, submerged perceptions, memories, and imaginations may surface. In a truly well-ordered society, every capable individual has a voice; likewise, in a sane and normally original mind, every valuable thought is welcomed into consciousness, even when it does not serve immediate self-preservative aims. In such minds, originality is not the symptom of disorder, but the highest expression of harmony between truth, freedom, and human growth.

It is difficult to attain the equilibrium of the intellectual functions, but exceedingly easy to lose it.

Common Sense, Science, and Speculation

Common sense treats all knowledge as simple and self-evident. It is satisfied with what appears obvious, with superficial and often tautological proofs. It distrusts theory, considering it fictitious or unreal, and regards sense data as ultimate, indisputable, universally valid, and independent of time and place.

Speculation represents the opposite extreme. It tends to view all knowledge—even axioms and the data of the senses—as complicated and perpetually in need of proof. It discovers difficulties and mysteries everywhere, even where none exist. No amount of evidence ever fully satisfies it. It often assigns theoretical considerations, or even negligible factors, as much importance as, or more importance than, practical realities. It continually postpones the boundary between facts and inferences, between data and hypotheses, pushing this threshold endlessly into the distance.

Between these two extremes—between the crude common sense of the plain man or the materialistic simplifier, and the unrestrained speculation of academic or sensational philosophy—stands science and philosophically disciplined common sense. This middle position assigns proportional weight to theory and practice and strives to distinguish clearly between fact and inference, certainty and probability.

Mental normality, in its ideal sense, belongs only to a privileged minority of talented individuals. Even in them it prevails only for a limited portion of life—during maturity—and even then only during waking, purposeful activity, excluding sleep, reverie, and exhaustion.

A man is not abnormal merely because he fails to adapt himself smoothly to continually changing and often contradictory circumstances. Adaptation to constant uncertainty would require a dulling of sensitivity and a regression toward brutality. A truly normal man would rather perish than accept such a regressive adaptation.

Since human society is not yet organized to reward genuine merit, an ambitious, fame-seeking genius must be regarded as less adapted than a wise, unambitious genius. And since reason appeared late in human evolution—since the human soul is younger than the human body—bodily adaptation is common, while psychical adaptation remains the privilege of the few. Agreement with the majority is therefore no test of mental normality. The majority may be sane in perception, but sound reasoning and conceptual clarity are still confined to a minority.

Animals are bodily better adapted than humans, but humans surpass animals psychically. Bodily adaptation fits only actual, present conditions, whereas psychical adaptation prepares for future and possible circumstances.

Primitive races, owing to physiological conditions such as pigmentation that protects against excessive heat, may be bodily better adapted than so-called higher races. Philistines, through muscular development, may be physically better adapted than men of genius. Yet psychical adaptation more than compensates for deficiencies in bodily adjustment.

The philistine concentrates nearly all vital energy on bodily preservation and reproduction, while the superior individual directs much of his energy toward intellectual and moral creation. Hence the former can endure physical strain, humiliation, monotony, and insecurity with relative insensibility and thus clings more easily to the existing social disorder. His method of preserving himself is regressive: he sacrifices sensitivity and higher aspiration. Parallel to this, he attempts to preserve the race by excessive reproduction, while the pseudo-superior leader—spokesman of parasitic minorities—encourages this course and denounces what he calls "race suicide." By this he attacks the superior individual's effort to preserve and elevate humanity by producing fewer but stronger, better-prepared human beings capable of resisting exploitation and injustice.

Instinct, Idea, and Adaptation

An idea, a sentiment, or a conscious reaction stands to an instinct or habit as an adventitious organ stands to a permanent one. Ideas arise from temporary surpluses of mental energy; instincts draw from stable reserves. Instincts are permanent psychical organs activated by recurring conditions, whereas ideas are temporary structures formed under novel pressures. Adaptation to society proceeds in two ways: imitation or invention. Imitation—doing what others do and suppressing individuality—is easier and has become instinctive. Invention—winning sympathy for new ways of acting—requires greater mental energy and remains an exceptional function, found chiefly in geniuses and in the mentally disordered.

Mysticism

In the mystic's brain, the insulation of nervous processes appears weakened. Mental currents short-circuit: where the normal mind maintains distinctions, the mystic fuses ideas. Concepts are stretched until they attempt to include everything, and in doing so they burst and become empty—pure extension without meaning.

At the summit of abstraction, mystics and idealistic philosophers often experience intellectual dizziness. They lose orientation and fail to return to the concrete world. Even when they descend again to facts, the confusion frequently persists.

Not every combination of words expresses a thought, nor does every grammatical question correspond to a logical one. Genuine questions arise when ideas are disconnected from their proper context or not yet integrated. Empty verbal questions mislead only the intellectually timid. Their emergence signals mental disequilibrium: language overpowers thought, form dethrones reason, and mysticism begins to rule.

Mathematical Mysticism

Many mathematical paradoxes arise from mistaking abstractions for reality. We simplify reality for convenience—speaking of moving points, instantaneous velocities, or statistical averages. Forgetting their symbolic nature, we treat them as real entities. Thus arise puzzles such as Zeno's paradoxes. A point, having no extension, cannot truly move, nor can an abstraction possess real existence. Another source of error lies in ignoring that qualitative change accompanies quantitative change. An angle vanishes when its sides vanish; continuity and simplicity dissolve under closer scrutiny. Mathematical perfection is first a product of imperfect perception and only secondarily an ideal construct.

Mysticism, whether religious or mathematical, is not a higher light but a twilight. It is either the dawn of original thought or the decline of clear thinking—the beginning of inquiry or the end of logic. It marks either the emergence of new understanding or a relapse into primitive confusion that sees relations everywhere or nowhere at all.

In this fragile balance between common sense, science, and speculation lies the measure of mental normality. When equilibrium is preserved, knowledge advances; when it is lost, thought dissolves into superstition or sterile abstraction.

The early conceptions of primitive thinkers—animism, the hypothesis of the soul, metempsychosis (reincarnation or migration of souls), Karma (Moera, Fate), mind-cure, and similar doctrines—were undoubtedly manifestations of progressive mystical thinking. They represented the first crude, groping attempts to extend old, materialistic and anthropomorphic explanations, and to graft upon them new hypotheses in order to account for newly and dimly perceived realities: the unity of man with Nature, the peculiar world of dreams, atavistic heredity, the chain of causal sequences, the influence of suggestion and of the mind upon the body, and related phenomena.

The revival of these same crude beliefs and practices in modern times, however—under new names and disguised in the scientific garb of more advanced hypotheses, as in spiritism, theosophy, Christian Science, and similar movements—must be regarded as a manifestation of regressive mysticism: a sign of decaying intelligence in the adherents and of sordid humbug in the leaders.

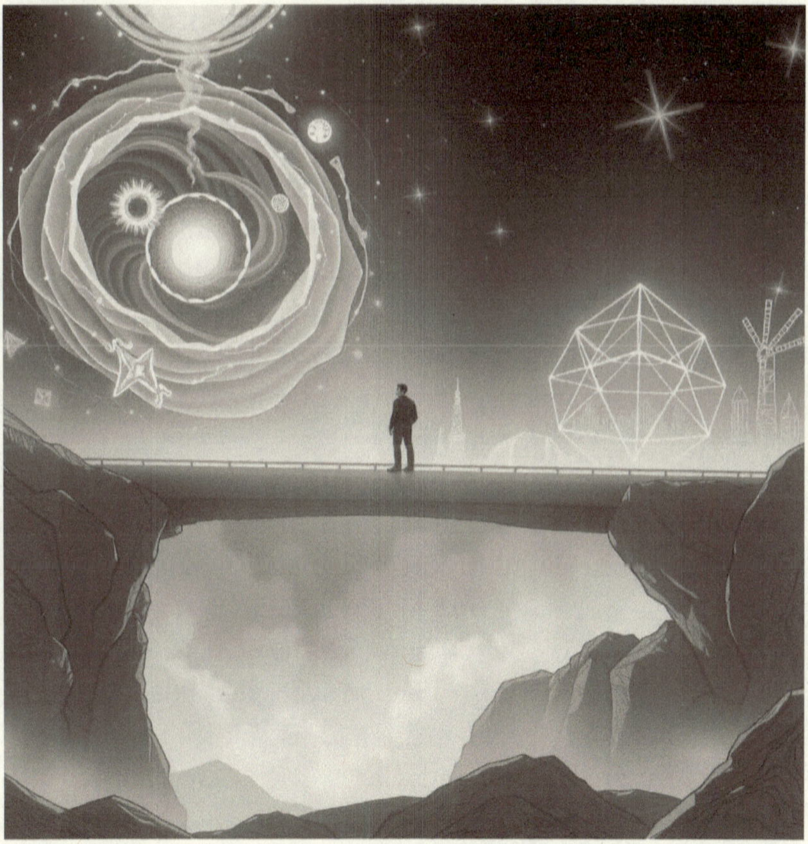

Mental laziness, incapacity, and impotence aspire to the possession of knowledge without intellectual effort, through so-called revelation, inspiration, intuition, dialectics, speculation, mystical or occult channels, or communion with spirits. Such minds lack patience for the laborious acquisition of knowledge through observation, experimentation, comparison, analysis, synthesis of sense data, and sustained reflection. Likewise, the intellectually dishonest prefer to dwell in the misty and obscure regions of verbal speculation, where their tricks and ignorance are less easily detected than in the clear light of honest, scientific investigation.

This intellectual parasitism—this dishonesty, laziness, impulsiveness, and incapacity for patient observation and clear, coherent, logical thinking; this craving for ready-made spiritual wealth, supernatural knowledge, and effortless power over Nature—has its exact analogue in the economic world. There, financial gambling and speculation replace productive labor, as both degenerate predatory classes and hopelessly struggling pariahs seek to become rich quickly, to seize ready-made wealth from others, and to acquire power without the ability or patience to create, produce, and accumulate gradually and securely.

Knowledge of the abstract, unknown, psychical, intangible, general, and dynamical begins by being almost identical with knowledge of the concrete, physical, tangible, and particular. It is then grasped by analogy, and finally becomes independent of such analogies. The nebulous and unstable thinker, after momentarily reaching this third stage, usually relapses into the second stage of analogy, and finally into the first stage of crude concretization and personification. He ends by speaking trivialities, commonplace truths, or even puerilities in abstract philosophical language; by treating ideas and feelings as if they were things, imaginary entities as if they were real, scientific laws as if they were external forces, relations as if they were facts, and concepts as if they were percepts—confusing related ideas with identical ones, and identical ones with unrelated.

Regressive Genius

Abilities that are declining in the course of human evolution—such as muscular strength, non-voluntary imitation, or pictorial thinking—when found in an extraordinary degree in an individual, may be regarded as forms of retrogressive genius. Such cases include extreme athletes, acrobats, certain actors, spiritistic mediums, or calculating prodigies who rely on vivid mental imagery. Thus, the poet's concrete, archaic, personification-laden language, when used for thought expression, indicates a more primitive and emotionally regressive mode of thinking, even while it may express a highly intellectualized and complex emotional life. Similarly, the exaggerated gestures, grimaces, and bodily mimicry of the actor reflect a more primitive and undifferentiated form of feeling and artistic expression, while at the same time representing a more advanced, socialized substitute for brute conflict, fighting, or violence.

Psychic Poison

The psychic organism, like the physiological one, harbors both harmful and harmless microbes. There exists a psychical self-poisoning analogous to physical intoxication, arising from the incomplete elimination of useless, indigestible, absurd, contradictory, or superfluous ideas. Our intellectual atmosphere, like our physical one, is polluted by mental waste: pseudo-concepts, still-born ideas, and intellectual refuse produced by degenerate or pseudo-geniuses. Ideas that cannot be assimilated or eliminated cause a form of mental constipation no less harmful than bodily disorders.

A healthy body craves food that maintains or restores equilibrium; a degenerated body longs for intoxicating or stupefying substances that yield momentary pleasure but hasten decay. Likewise, a healthy mind craves clear knowledge, attainable truth, moderate emotion, and reality; a degenerated mind seeks intoxication, ecstasy, insoluble problems, violent emotions, illusions, and mystical excitement.

Just as producers and dealers of alcohol recruit their consumers chiefly from those to whom a plain, orderly life is inaccessible or distasteful, so pseudo-philosophers, pseudo-prophets, and mystical writers recruit their admirers from those to whom plain truth is unattainable or insufficiently stimulating.

These producers of psychic intoxicants appear more influential than they truly are because of their noise, obtrusiveness, and self-proclaimed importance.

While many artistic and literary aberrations harm only limited circles of similarly degenerate minds, there exists a far more dangerous class of morally perverted individuals who manufacture mental narcotics for the masses. In exchange for salaries or privileges granted by exploiters, they distribute these intoxicants under the guise of official religion, public education, patriotic rhetoric, political leadership, sensational news, or compulsory enthusiasm for sports and spectacles. These mental narcotics—dispensed from pulpit, platform, classroom, and press under the cloak of respectability—are more destructive than alcohol itself, for they paralyze critical judgment, maintain submission, and perpetuate ignorance.

What narcotics are more enduringly mind-deadening than the worship of patriotic fetishes, national self-conceit, empty slogans such as "constitution" or "liberty," the false hopes fostered by pseudo-rulers, the magical threats and promises of priesthoods, the adulterated historical instruction of schools, the theological nonsense forced upon undeveloped minds, the distortion of free thought, and the fraudulent sensationalism of the press? These poisons do not merely intoxicate; they arrest the intellectual and moral progress of mankind.

In this sense, regressive mysticism and intellectual dishonesty represent not harmless eccentricities, but grave dangers to human development. Only clear thinking, disciplined inquiry, and moral courage can protect the mind from such slow and subtle forms of decay.

Sex and Mental Superiority.— Women are, as a rule, born philistines in the sense that they lack enduring intellectual needs and sustained ideal or moral aspirations. Social gallantry—an invention of idle, parasitical, and sensual men—encourages them to persist in this state of mental inertia. Intellectual activity appears as a relatively permanent, organic, and primary function in men—owing to physiological factors not yet fully understood and to the constant pressure of the struggle for life, competition, and responsibility—whereas in women it appears as an occasional, intermittent, and secondary function. From this difference arise greater disharmony, instability, exhaustion, and compensatory deficiencies in women than in men. Hence superior men tend to be more many-sided, more balanced, and more consistent with their sex than superior women. After the end of formal education and the cessation of the stimuli of sexual selection, more women than men relapse into philistinism, conservatism, emotionalism, superstition, and narrow, prosaic pursuits. Knowledge and truth thus remain, for women, a means to success rather than an end in themselves.

In women, reason and the love of truth are intermittent and unstable, remaining largely theoretical. Abstract principles, logical consistency, and disinterested sentiments rarely guide their conduct, which flows instead from self-interest, instinct, shifting emotions, habit, suggestion from acknowledged or self-appointed authorities, and imitation of outward forms. A woman may invoke reason or philosophy to inspire admiration in intellectual men, to depreciate unattainable possessions, to criticize another woman's conduct, or to justify her own past actions; yet in her personal affairs she rarely appeals to such principles. An intelligent man, once committed to a life companion, generally ceases to seek further conquests; even intelligent married women, however, often continue to pursue admiration from men without clear purpose. Of moral and disinterested sentiments, woman is said to possess chiefly condescending pity toward bodily and social inferiors—focused on palpable physical suffering—and maternal altruism. She is portrayed as lacking a sense of justice, impersonal duty, constant and disinterested friendship, and a higher altruism embracing all classes, nations, and races. Maternal altruism is thus considered her principal ennobling trait. In religion she seeks self-preservation rather than metaphysical or cosmical understanding. Intellectual functions in women remain subordinated to, and undifferentiated from, self-preservative and reproductive instincts.

Love affairs, particularly for the socially parasitic woman, are not merely sexual relations but sources of intellectual gratification, vanity, relief from ennui, power over others, self-valuation, and social advancement—often serving as a means of approaching prominent or superior men through sexual attraction. To woman, a love affair tends to constitute the whole of life; to man, it is one episode among many. Even intellectually inclined women often engage in higher pursuits from affection for a particular man or in the hope of admiration, thereby subordinating intellectual achievement to sexual or material aims. When women participate in frivolous or coarse talk, it is attributed not to sensuality but to a perceived competence in one of the few domains—aside from adornment—where they believe themselves entitled to speak. The so-called "free-loving" women, described as possessing masculine sensuality, are said rarely to bear children and thus cannot perpetuate their type. Because women expect from love a range of satisfactions rarely fulfilled by one individual, they are portrayed as more dissatisfied with marriage than men and as lacking "soul chastity," remaining mentally polygamous while physically monogamous.

If theories of sex inheritance that deny strict paternal-to-son and maternal-to-daughter transmission are accepted, then woman's intellectual inferiority is interpreted as constitutional and physiological rather than social. Differences in upbringing and social condition are then viewed not as causes but as effects of this inferiority. Physical strength is regarded as a negligible factor in shaping relations between the sexes, and oppression alone is held insufficient to extinguish intelligence. Since manifestations of women's intellect are deemed inferior across fields, even in traditionally feminine occupations, this is taken as further evidence of a physiological foundation. Observations that periods of social stress yield a higher proportion of male births are cited as corroboration. Superior women are therefore described as abnormal, exhibiting greater disharmony between intellect and instinct than male geniuses.

Women are thus said to combine the empty-mindedness of philistine men with the affectation of pseudo-superior men, without possessing the latter's embryonic superiority. In random comparison, the female group is portrayed as clustering closely around the philistine level, showing little mental variability, whereas the male group spreads across a wide range—from genius and talent through mediocrity to weakness and insanity—displaying greater diversity above and below the philistine norm.

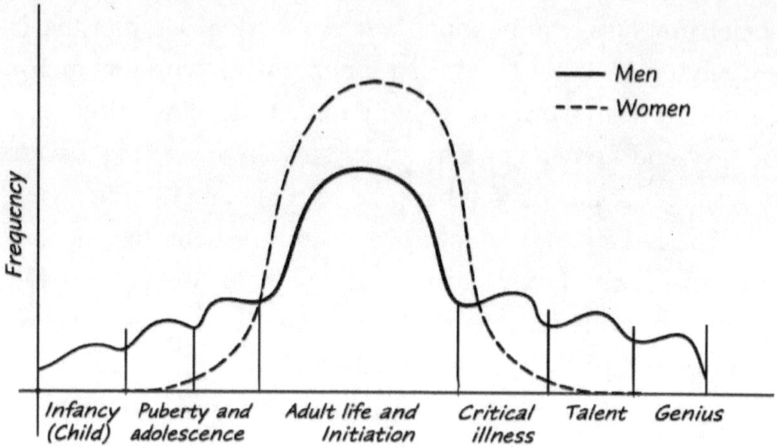

Or, more precisely, if we represent the different mental states as distinct arcs of a circle, and indicate their frequency by measuring along the radius, the result may be expressed in the form of the following diagram:

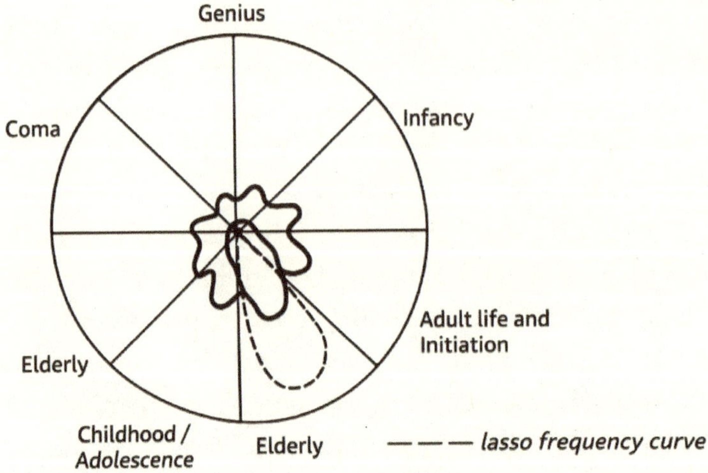

Women, as a rule, are born philistines: their intellectual needs remain rudimentary. They continue to consult fortune-tellers, clairvoyants, and similar figures; they persist in identifying the church with religion itself, titles with merit, and outward position with inner worth—even when they are educated in colleges and live among intellectual men. Men, by contrast, are generally made philistines by circumstances—by social pressure, exploitation, and oppression. Despite the most stupefying drudgery imposed upon them, working men still gather to hear words of enlightenment; despite abject misery, hungry and homeless tramps may be seen devouring a scrap of newspaper or a book that happens to come into their hands.

The female individual appears to represent an older, more primitive form of living being than the male. More precisely, the most primitive form of life—the parthenogenetic, hermaphroditic, or self-reproductive organism—branched off at an early period, when bodily progress predominated over psychical progress, into female individuals that remained closer to this original type, and into male individuals endowed with fewer racial or instinctive traits but greater capacity to inherit acquired characteristics, more energy, greater variability, and higher adaptability. The male's role was at first merely to stimulate reproduction; later it became contributory. It may be inferred that when the female engages in sexual intercourse without attraction or love for the male, his role remains merely stimulating and not genuinely cooperative.

If the female inherits and, like the child, recapitulates organized, racial, primitive characteristics, but not the more recent functional variations, we can understand her tendency toward superstition, conservatism, mental confusion, irritability, impulsiveness, intolerance, despotism, vindictiveness, and unsociability; and we can also understand why, despite protection from the uncertainties of the struggle for life, she may still display greed, deceit, envy, untruthfulness, selfishness, intellectual inertia, craving for power and caste distinction, and incapacity for disinterested friendship. From this standpoint it becomes intelligible why the progress of woman lags behind that of man, and why higher aspirations are not readily inherited by her, since such aspirations do not easily become a common property of the species.

Man is destined to supply woman with the necessities of life; but for woman to become progressive, progress itself must pass from the possession of a few or of a privileged class into the possession of all. Woman's progress normally comes through custom and practice, not spontaneously nor through direct intellectual assimilation from the complex social environment. Her normal originality has hitherto lacked both the strength and the opportunity to be exposed to, and to resist, the inert currents and pressures emanating from the surrounding world. Creative originality has therefore remained largely a male attribute, and only exceptionally the attribute of geniuses standing nearest the periphery of the struggling human mass; it has rarely become the property of women except where prolonged usefulness, training, or social and physiological inheritance has made it possible. Paramnesia.—In paramnesia, one mistakes an actual perception, thought, recollection—and one may add, emotion—for a past one; with every new experience the patient feels as though it had been experienced before. This sense of a "before," however, is not wholly a fabrication of the mind. A very recent moment is mistaken for a remote and indefinite past because attention, being distracted or absorbed, gives so little hold to present experiences that they do not persist clearly in memory, nor become firmly linked with other experiences. The persons and objects before the eyes, the events occurring in one's presence, receive so little attention—consciousness being absorbed by organic sensations, inner experiences, reverie, or conceptual thinking—that they easily fall out of awareness, or rather out of marginal consciousness, only to be brought back again through their persistence or recurrence.

Recollections of very remote experiences are ordinarily vague. The paramnesiac therefore infers unconsciously, from the vagueness of recollection—caused by incomplete and inattentive perception—that the experience belongs to a distant past. In reality, the experience is present, or intermittently renewed, instead of being continuously retained, as it is in a normally attentive and unpreoccupied mind.

I am inclined to think that a slight degree of paramnesia is a familiar experience even to well-balanced thinkers—to men who are often deeply, though not hypnotically, absorbed in following long chains of thought and reasoning. While such men are mentally engaged, they must constantly repress recurring perceptions that attempt to seize their attention; they must struggle against the emotions aroused by these perceptions and against the associated trains of thought. Only those who become totally absorbed in their inner processes—whose perceptive centers are, as it were, completely shut while inner activity is in progress—or those who never pursue any thought far or seriously, who rarely have ideas awakened by remote or past impressions, and especially those who restrict their mental life to mere perception, to passive looking-on without interpretation or reflection—only such people are free from paramnesic illusions.

The superior man's continual inner activity—his habitual absorption in conceptual thinking—draws heavily upon the energy of the immediately lower brain functions, such as active memory and active perception or observation. In addition, his incipient centrifugal, outward-directed or motor currents often overflow into centripetal, inward-directed or sensory channels. For this reason his perception becomes functionally or temporarily obtuse and sluggish. It is not so much passive reception as active interpretation that suffers. While absorbed, he may see and hear, yet fail to understand what he sees and hears, because he is occupied with digesting, assimilating, and correlating the experiences, impressions, and teachings of the past. What is commonly called the genius's paramnesia, amnesia, forgetfulness, or absent-mindedness simply means that impressions perceived imperfectly, slowly, or inattentively cannot be remembered with the same clarity as impressions received when the mind is unoccupied, receptive, and ready to absorb whatever presents itself.

To regard, with Lombroso, the genius's absent-mindedness or temporary incapacity for receiving new impressions while he is digesting old ones as a sign of degeneration or abnormality; to see pathology in his inability to attend simultaneously to details and to wholes, to immediate ends and to remote aims; to interpret as defects his tactlessness—his inability to pursue truth and justice while at the same time ingratiating himself with truth-hating, parasitic elites; his unsociability—his inability to meditate deeply and yet enjoy the company of frivolous, thoughtless philistines; his unadaptedness—his refusal to conform to obsolete orders, beaten paths, empty conventions, or to bow before monarchs and other drones while preparing the way for a more just, democratic social order—this, in short, is as absurd as reproaching a man for being unable to eat new food while his stomach is already full, for not being in two places at once, or for failing to focus his eyes simultaneously on near and distant objects.

It is far more reasonable to see degeneracy, abnormality, or at best arrested development in the pseudo-superior man's one-sidedness and in the philistine's incapacity to rise above mere suggestibility and passive perception; in his inability to compare, harmonize, or discard the contradictory and empty beliefs imposed upon him by his various exploiters; in his blindness to the inconsistency between his professed opinions and his actual conduct. To interpret the superior man's contempt for, and lack of skill in, philistine pursuits—such as submissiveness, blind imitation, mental passivity, worship of brute strength, of material success, of mere size and quantity, the pursuit of comfort and wealth as ends in themselves, compliance with fashion and convention, degrading hero-worship, and reliance on external saviors, gods, leaders, or quacks—as signs of inferiority or maladjustment is as irrational as calling man a degenerate animal because he is weaker than his animal relatives in muscular strength, speed, or sensory acuity.

What need has man to rival animals in physical prowess when he can invent tools, machines, and weapons, and when his intellect can summon the hidden forces of nature and compel them to work on his behalf? Yet just as it would be foolish to discard the oil lamp entirely because gas and electric light exist, so it would be unwise to neglect bodily strength altogether. It is only futile to strive after the agility of apes when far superior means lie within reach.

The genius rejects philistine paths because, when followed blindly beyond the crossroads, they lead only to blind alleys. He too begins by traveling along these paths, but he abandons them as soon as he discovers broader roads leading forward and upward. Still more absurd is the tendency to brand as abnormal not only the superior man's differences from the average, but even his sharing in common human weaknesses—such as vanity (though he has more reason than most to feel pride), or inconsistency (as though any man, especially one whose intellect continually outruns his instincts, habits, and environment, could be entirely free from it).

Since the genius—or the precursor of the truly higher human being, who will be the exact opposite of Nietzsche's confused, capitalistic fantasy of a brutal, egotistic, antisocial, predatory "super-man"—necessarily springs from philistine ancestry, and is nothing more than a more freely, harmoniously, and many-sidedly developed human being, it cannot reasonably be expected that he should differ entirely from ordinary mortals or that he should retain and employ all their lower capacities in addition to his higher ones.

What has been said about the genius's apparent mental deficiencies accompanying deep inner absorption applies equally to the nervous disturbances that often follow intense or prolonged intellectual labor. If geniuses suffer from nervous exhaustion, mental depression, lowered vitality, melancholia, or epileptic seizures; if many of them eventually break down or even lose their mental balance under the combined burden of sustained intellectual effort and social prejudice, ostracism, ridicule, adverse circumstances, or persecution—what does this prove? It proves only that one cannot both spend and retain one's energy; that sustained work necessarily brings fatigue; that even an intellectual giant must pay a price when he overtaxes his strength; that even geniuses are not immune to social disapproval; and that pioneering labor is inevitably surrounded by danger. It proves nothing whatever in favor of the notion that genius and degeneration, or intellectual creation and epileptic convulsions, are equivalent. Such a conclusion would be as absurd as asserting that energy is identical with the fatigue or weakness that follows its expenditure.

The genius takes delight in testing and exercising his intellectual power, his capacity for original thought and sustained mental effort, and is therefore inclined to overestimate—and thus overstrain—his own resources. In this respect he resembles the athlete, who is merely a more brutal, more primitive, and therefore more robust type of philistine. The athlete takes such pleasure in feeling his muscular strength and dexterity that he frequently attempts the impossible and thus exposes himself to accidents. The ordinary philistine, on the other hand, is largely spared both bodily and mental self-inflicted injuries, because his instinct of self-preservation prevents him from attempting what he senses he cannot accomplish. His misoneism is not, as Lombroso—the originator of the term—was inclined to believe, an aversion to all change or novelty as such. It is rather an aversion to mental exertion and to original, unconventional thinking, rooted in his incapacity for such effort and guided by a fundamentally healthy instinct of self-protection.

The End

www.ingramcontent.com/pod-product-compliance
Lightning Source LLC
LaVergne TN
LVHW100724061126
851857LV00011B/387
* 9 7 8 9 3 7 2 4 4 1 7 4 1 *

Günther Ossimitz

Entwicklung systemischen Denkens

Klagenfurter Beiträge zur Didaktik der Mathematik

Band 1